# USING OCCUPATIONAL THERAPY MODELS IN PRACTICE

*Commissioning Editor:* Rita Demetriou-Swanwick
*Development Editor:* Catherine Jackson
*Project Manager:* Kiruthiga Kasthuriswamy
*Designer:* Stewart Larking
*Illustration Manager:* Merlyn Harvey
*Illustrator:* Ethan Danielson

# USING OCCUPATIONAL THERAPY MODELS IN PRACTICE A FIELD GUIDE

**Merrill Turpin** B.Occ.Thy., Grad Dip Counsel., & PhD
Lecturer, Division of occupational therapy,
School of Health and Rehabilitation Sciences,
The University of Queensland, Brisbane, Australia

**Michael K. Iwama** PhD, MSc, BSc, BScOT, OT(C)
Associate Professor, Graduate Department of Rehabilitation
Sciences, and Department of Occupational Science and
Occupational Therapy, Faculty of Medicine,
University of Toronto, Toronto, Canada

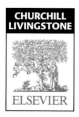

CHURCHILL
LIVINGSTONE

ELSEVIER

EDINBURGH  LONDON  NEW YORK  OXFORD  PHILADELPHIA  ST LOUIS
SYDNEY  TORONTO 2011

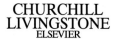
CHURCHILL
LIVINGSTONE
ELSEVIER

© 2011 Elsevier Ltd. All rights reserved.

ISBN 978 0 7234 3494 8

**British Library Cataloguing in Publication Data**
A catalogue record for this book is available from the British Library

**Library of Congress Cataloging in Publication Data**
A catalog record for this book is available from the Library of Congress

### Notices

ELSEVIER   your source for books,
journals and multimedia
in the health sciences
**www.elsevierhealth.com**

Working together to grow
libraries in developing countries

www.elsevier.com | www.bookaid.org | www.sabre.org

ELSEVIER   BOOK AID International   Sabre Foundation

The
Publisher's
policy is to use
paper manufactured
from sustainable forests

Printed in China

# CONTENTS

# PREFACE

As occupational therapy forges ahead into its second century, the time seemed right to take stock of its current approach to theory and practice. Over the last century, much has changed in this great profession in terms of its ideas and practices. The industrialized world has moved from a period of modernity that favoured singular, positivist explanations of human phenomena and truth, to a post-modern condition marked by plural and relative views of truth and the world around us. The primacy and meanings of 'doing' in contemporary occupational therapy interpreted through the lens of the rational individual is being challenged and expanded to include the possibilities that come with diverse views of truth and collective experience. What was once a biomedically dominated body of theory and knowledge is expanding into the realms of critical social science and social justice. Many of these alterations have been prompted by changes in the greater contexts within which occupational therapy ideas and practices have existed. The evolution of our ideas and theory attest to the enduring occupational therapy belief that humans carry enormous capacity to adapt to diverse environments and their varying circumstances.

As much as these changes present enormous challenges for the occupational therapy scholar and theorist who must find a way to explain the phenomena and shared experiences around 'doing', the challenges for occupational therapy students and practitioners to comprehend and navigate the occupational therapy theory to practise continuum across a landscape of diverse contexts of daily life and practice has to be an even more daunting one. Thus, the authors, who have practised and taught occupational therapy theory for over half a century combined, saw the need for a different kind of textbook on occupational therapy models.

What was needed was a textbook that presented a uniform overview of the more popular models of the profession, and one that was written from the perspectives of *practice* and the *practitioner*. We heard and empathized with many practising occupational therapists around the world who were feeling disrespected and shut out of the science and theoretical discourses of their profession. To make matters worse, therapists were feeling inadequately prepared to take theories and imperatives for practice that were thought up and theorized in locations far removed from the proving grounds of practice. What was really needed in occupational therapy education and practice was a useful resource that students and practitioners could take into and use within varying contexts of the occupational therapy practice arena, with the endorsement that they could, and should, make the necessary connection between theory and what actually takes place in that crucial dynamic uniting client and therapist. The need to support our colleagues in the field to use theory to help their clients solve the challenges of day to day living led to the infusion of *clinical (professional) reasoning* into the material.

In addition, the authors recognized a need for a book on occupational therapy theory that would take into account the emerging challenge that culture presented to occupational therapy practice in a global world. More and more, occupational therapists around the world have come to recognize the challenges and limitations of taking certain (singular and universal) explanations of occupation and occupational therapy (which Iwama contends would reflect and favour the cultural norms of a model's origins) across cultural boundaries of meaning. This evolving discourse on culture and theory would also reveal the structural issues of power intertwined in the client, therapist and institution dynamic, affecting how practitioners reconcile what they want to do, and how they will do, with their clients. Instead of merely conveying instructions on how a particular model should be applied, a new kind of theory resource that would aim to empower and enable the therapist to critically understand models and how to judiciously select and apply them, was required. With such ideas and tensions in mind, and while the authors contemplated their various needs in occupational therapy theory classes in Australia, North America, the UK and Europe, Asia, South America and Africa, the basic framework and content of this book you are now examining was born.

While not claiming to be a historical document, this book places those theoretical frameworks that aim to guide practice into a broader historical and situational context. Ideas and practices are located in time and space. They exist within a historical context in which they follow on from what has come before and they pave the way for what might come in the future. They also sprout from the fertile soil of other ideas and practices that surround them, both locally and more broadly. As a profession where theory and practice are intimately linked, occupational therapy has a rich tradition of developing conceptual models that aim to guide practice. However, these models of practice also form part of a century-old development of ideas and practices. We believe that no single model is adequate and universally applicable in all occupational therapy situations. Each model is profoundly complex and represents a constellation of conditions, truisms, ideals, cultural norms and values that preceded and now surround them. A similar dance between a model and the contexts of conditions and ideas that contributed to its current form occurs between the model and the unique experiences and circumstances of daily life of the client. The reasoning occupational therapist is the mediator who strives to bring the best and safest fit between the client and what occupational therapy can offer.

This book provides a small window into the progress of theory and practice over the three decades from the 1980s by presenting nine current occupational therapy models and a review of their historical development. In a rapidly changing world, it is easy to lose sight of what had led up to the current situation and to only look towards the future. However, in doing so, we risk losing important ideas that might have temporarily been put aside in favour of ones that meet current challenges. We hope that this book will assist occupational therapists to review some of the ideas that have been important over the past three decades and to 'dust them off', look at them anew and determine their utility in the current context.

[Merrill] The writing of this book also has its own history. The seeds of its development grew out of an invitation from the Division of Occupational Therapy at The University of Queensland to Professor Michael Iwama to become an adjunct professor. His acceptance of this position provided the opportunity for the forging of many important professional relationships for occupational therapy staff members at The University of Queensland. This book is the result of one such association (but only one of many). I wish to thank Michael for being a great collaborator, for encouraging me to see the value in many of my ideas, and for sharing his wealth of experience and breadth of vision for occupational therapy.

[Michael] I remember how blessed and fortunate I felt when I arrived at The University of Queensland in 2003 to begin this wonderful association with the occupational therapists of Australia. I was stunned & impressed by the highly experienced, learned and capable academic team there. I was most impressed in particular by an emerging light in our profession by the name of Merrill Turpin. Though I was initially invited to share ideas about culture and theory in OT with my Australian colleagues, I ended up being schooled by Dr Turpin on these subjects. As you read through this text, you will readily appreciate that the majority of content is Merrill Turpin's. It has been a privilege to 'piggy-back' on Dr Turpin's ideas and work, to be inspired and to be allowed to partner with her in bringing this resource to the classrooms and practice arenas of our great profession.

We hope that this book will ultimately be the useful resource to students, practitioners and educators that we envisioned. And if knowledge is indeed power, we would like to see that power, customarily ceded to theoretical side of the continuum, transferred to and vetted in the crucible of occupational therapy practice. We hope that in turn, over time, therapists will once again be regarded as the holders of the essence and potential power of occupational therapy. Occupational therapy models should be interpreted and understood through the lens of practice and in the daily life experiences of our clients. Models should ultimately be evaluated by their usefulness in exacting positive change and benefit to its clients and service recipients. Therefore, we hope that the practising occupational therapist will utilize this book in a different way than they might have with previous theory books. We hope that the student and therapist will bring the book into their places of study and work where it can be handily and conveniently referred to, within the domain of occupational therapy practice.

# ACKNOWLEDGEMENTS

We both have families whose love and support have sustained us through the long but enjoyable time of writing the manuscript. I (Merrill) would like to thank my husband Iain Renton for providing the drawing of the window for the book. And I (Michael) would like to thank my wife Sharon for her enduing patience with my obsession for my profession. We would also like to thank Catherine Jackson, the development editor of the book, who provided gentle and understanding guidance and for whose patience and professionalism we are very appreciative.

Merrill Turpin & Michael Iwama
Brisbane, Australia and Toronto, Canada 2010

# Introduction

*The aspects of things that are most important for use are hidden because of their simplicity and familiarity.*

Ludwig Wittgenstein

This book is about the practice of occupational therapy. It is about the process that occupational therapists, as professionals, use to make decisions about professional action. It is also about the ideas that are (or have been) put together into structured frameworks in order to guide the practice of occupational therapy. In the quote above, Ludwig Wittgenstein alluded to the invisibility that occurs when ideas become so accepted by a community that they are no longer noticed or commented upon. Phenomenologists refer to this situation as the *natural attitude*, whereby we can be unaware of the assumptions that shape our perspectives. In the professional realm, developing conceptual frameworks is valuable because they help us to be aware of many of the assumptions that are so central to our profession but often go unnoticed.

Occupational therapists have a well-developed practice of using conceptual frameworks to make explicit the ideas (and their relationships) that form the basis of their practice. The impetus for this might come partly from the fact that much of occupational therapy practice occurs within the context of ordinary daily life. As this can make the occupational therapy knowledge base appear like 'common sense' to many, occupational therapy might need to clarify the unique nature of its perspective. Conceptual frameworks assist us to demonstrate that our knowledge base isn't just common sense. The fact that occupational therapists are sought and accepted in society and able to provide services that others cannot, suggests that occupational therapy knowledge might better be described as 'uncommon sense'. Occupational therapy frameworks, which we will call models throughout this book, are useful for exploring our profession's uncommon sense.

© 2011 Elsevier Ltd.
DOI: 10.1016/B978-07234-3494-8.00009-7

1

As professionals, occupational therapists wrestle in their daily working lives with the complexities of facilitating the occupational performance of clients or populations. Occupational therapists know that it is very difficult to identify generalized principles about what helps people to do what they need and want to in their daily lives. This is because so many factors influence this outcome. They know that individuals, who vary considerably in their nature, abilities and interests, live their lives in very specific contexts. They also know that these contexts are very complex – that they include people, places, materials and equipment, and have cultural, spatial and temporal dimensions.

Occupational therapists know that the way people think about and experience themselves is dependent upon their ability to participate in their specific life contexts. The requirements for participation in daily life are as varied as people themselves and their particular life circumstances. Such requirements might include being able to perform particular tasks for themselves or for others; performing tasks by themselves or with others; restraining from action in particular situations; and fulfilling the roles they expect of themselves or are expected by others in their 'group' and the broader society in which they live.

In this book, we propose that the central concern of occupational therapy is *facilitating context-dependent participation through occupation*. Two concepts are important in this core concern; context and participation through occupation. First, occupational therapy has always acknowledged the importance of the context in which people live and act to both living and action. People do particular things in particular places at particular historical and chronological times. Occupational therapy has generally used the term 'environment' to discuss context. Over time, the aspects of the environment that influence performance have been identified more specifically, as evident in the adjectives used, such as physical, social, societal, institutional, political, cultural, and temporal. Essentially, human occupation occurs in a particular time and place as well as having relevance to particular people and groups.

Second, occupational therapy aims to assist people to participate in ways that are meaningful to them in their local situations and broader societies. In common usage, the word participation means to take part or share in something. Many current views in occupational therapy assume that human occupation is the primary vehicle through which people take part or share in the communities in which they live their daily lives. They also know that, due to circumstances, people might have difficulty taking part in the daily lives of their communities, whether those communities be family or other social groups.

## A HISTORICAL AND CONTEXTUAL APPROACH

The decisions people make and the things they do often make sense if you understand the underlying contexts of their experiences. These experiences have temporal and spatial influences, that is, people live and act in particular places at particular times and in the context of their own biographical and social histories. Professions also exist within particular times and places and with a history that influences its ideas. How these ideas relate and resonate with current societal conditions, as well as those in the future, may determine the usefulness and viability of the profession.

In this book, we present nine conceptual frameworks, which we refer to as models of practice. We have chosen these models of practice because we believe they represent the major conceptual frameworks that are particular to occupational therapy (and therefore relevant to occupational therapy practice). As discussed in Chapter 1, terminology for conceptual frameworks in occupational therapy is inconsistent and, as occupational therapists use a wide range of knowledge from outside of the profession, much of this knowledge is not specific or unique to occupational therapy. Therefore we have not included conceptual or practice frameworks that occupational therapists might use in particular practice areas to provide detailed guidance about specific assessments and interventions (often referred to as frames of reference). Rather, by focusing on occupational therapy models of practice, we aim to overview and discuss the way occupational therapy theory and practice is conceptualized by a range of different authors in different parts of the world.

We have tried to capture how time and place might have influenced the ideas of particular occupational therapy authors by taking a historical approach to the models that we present. While a number of texts have done this by tracing some of the philosophical roots of the profession, our purpose in this book is to place occupational therapy practice models within the context of the ideas prevalent at the time and place in which they were developed. Some of the models we present have been updated in the context of several editions. Others were published at an earlier time and have not been updated. Regardless of when they were first (or last) published, the models in this book have been chosen because they encompass many of the important ideas that have shaped current occupational therapy perspectives. Many of the ideas presented in these conceptual models have become embedded within current occupational therapy philosophy and their influence on practice has been enduring. Presenting a range of models that have been developed over the past three decades (or so) of the profession will provide practitioners and theorists with a very condensed view of the ideas that have shaped the profession of occupational therapy. We hope that this book will encourage readers to ask how relevant and able to complement occupational therapy practice our models will be as the profession moves forward. By comprehending the influence of historical context on theory development, current and future occupational therapists may be compelled to critically consider the relevance and importance of occupational therapy, and contribute to the important processes of updating existing models and innovating new ones.

## WESTERN MODELS OF HEALTH

As many of the major occupational therapy models were developed in the context of Western views of health, we commence with a discussion of some of these ideas. Historically, occupational therapy has concentrated on the participation of *individuals*, because of its development as a profession in the Western world, particularly in the health sector with its individualistic and mechanistic understanding of health. In occupational therapy, this focus on individuals appears to be changing in line with the broader trends within health towards an increased concern for population health. We propose that three models of health have influenced occupational therapy practice models.

These are biomedical, biopsychosocial and socioecological models of health. (A range of different labels have been used for the last model including a social model of health. However, we have chosen not to use this term as it is often confused with a social model of disability, which is quite different.)

Reed (2005) and Kielhofner (2009) both identified four historical periods in occupational therapy's short history. These are outlined in Table I.1. Essentially, both of these classifications commence with a time when the ideas that became fundamental to occupational therapy were developed by other movements such as the Moral Treatment and Arts and Crafts movements. This time is followed by a period in which occupational therapists worked on the premise that productive and meaningful human action facilitated good health. The third period in occupational therapy's history was characterized by the dominance of the mechanistic view of humans that was prevalent in health towards the end of the twentieth century and the final period was described by both authors as a return to the profession's foundational principles. Whiteford et al. (2000) emphasized that, in this fourth period, occupational therapy was *returning* to a focus on occupation that had always been present in the profession, rather than developing a new direction. They referred to this reaffirmation of focus as a "renaissance of occupation" (p. 61).

These periods or paradigms align with trends in the broader context of health. The first trend in health during the periods outlined by Reed and Kielhofner was dominated by a conceptual framework frequently referred to as the *biomedical model of health*. This model gradually became the dominant model of health in Western countries from the mid-1800s through the rise of medicine. In discussing this model of health, Taylor and Field (2003) explained that the development of medicine is often described in terms of dramatic breakthroughs. They stated, "In this 'heroic' view of medicine, the struggle for better health is seen as a 'war' waged by doctors and medical scientists against an impersonal enemy called disease on the battleground of the human body" (p. 21). They listed the main assumptions of the biomedical model of health as:

- Health is the absence of biological abnormality
- Diseases have specific causes
- The human body is likened to a machine to be restored to health through personalised treatments that arrest, or reverse, the disease process
- The health of a society is seen as largely dependent on the state of medical knowledge and the availability of medical resources (pp. 21–22)

Taylor and Field (2003) explained that the dominance of the biomedical model of health was consolidated in the nineteenth and early twentieth centuries through the development of hospitals. The biomedical model is an expert model in which the patient is expected to submit (passively) to investigations of their bodies (directly or indirectly through medical technology such as X-ray and MRI) in order to locate the cause of their health problems.

Although occupational therapy always had humanistic influences as well as biomedical ones, the mechanistic ideas of the West are most evident in the period that both Reed and Kielhofner referred to as 'mechanistic' (because it was dominated by the *body-as-machine* metaphor) and in the occupational therapy models of the 1980s. These models emphasized the effect on performance

Table 1.1  *Periods in occupational therapy history*

| | Reed (2005) | | Kielhofner (2009) | | |
|---|---|---|---|---|---|
| Time | Period & influences | Characteristics | Time | Paradigm | Characteristics |
| 1800–1899 | Preformative period: Moral treatment movement, Arts & Crafts movement | Ideas from these movements led to occupational therapy practice in mental health institutions | 18th & 19th centuries | Moral treatment pre-paradigm | Participation in daily activities contributed to health |
| 1900–1929 | Formative period: Philosophy of pragmatism | Development of foundational terms and concepts | Beginning of 20th century (1900s) | Paradigm of occupation | Interrelatedness of mind, body and environment to engagement in occupation |
| 1930–1965 | Mechanistic period: Philosophy of medicine and scientific (quantitative) method | Many formative concepts "forgotten" & new concepts developed | Late 1940s & 1950s | Mechanistic paradigm | Focus on impairments in internal mechanisms–biomechanical, intrapsychic & neurological |
| 1966–present | Modern period: Return of formative ideas & acceptance of qualitative methods | Development of models of practice, extension of understanding of occupation in daily life | 1960s–present | Contemporary paradigm: return to occupation | Return to occupation, focus on factors that influence occupational performance |

of an individual's impairments, referred to as *performance components*. However, a contrasting humanistic concern for people *as people* remained a primary characteristic of occupational therapy, even when the influence of biomedicine was at its strongest. During this time, a biomedical understanding of people characterized by the body-as-machine metaphor was contrasted by an open systems understanding. An open systems approach conceptualizes humans as consisting of layers of mutually influencing systems. Psychological and social aspects of the human experience are considered along with biomedical concerns. A systems approach occurred concurrently, and is often associated with the biopsychosocial model of health, the second major health model that has influenced occupational therapy theory (and the one that characterizes occupational therapy most closely).

Western health systems embraced a biopsychosocial model of health in the latter part of the twentieth century. In 1977, George Engel published an article advocating for a model of health that went beyond an understanding of health that was limited to a normative view of the body and the absence of disease. He called it the biopsychosocial model. As the name suggests, the model acknowledged that biological, psychological and social aspects of a person's life influenced health. This model of health focused on well-being (which is more than just the absence of disease) and the subjective experience of health (rather than just the physical manifestations of disease). Over the course of time, a biopsychosocial approach became a dominant model for health, particularly in service organizations other than hospitals (where a biomedical model still predominates).

The subjective experience of ill-health and disability was a major health research focus in the early 1980s. Based in medical anthropology and known as the phenomenology of illness, research was undertaken that distinguished between disease and the experience of illness (e.g. see Good & DelVecchio Good, 1980; Toombs, 1992). This research demonstrated that the *experience* of ill-health is separate to, and often different from, disease. For example, a person might have the physical signs of a disease but feel quite well and others might experience ill-health and disability in the absence of physical signs. In the biopsychosocial model, a more holistic understanding of health was emphasized that included both the physical signs of heath and illness as well as subjective experience.

The individual is seen within the context of the broader systems in which the person lives. Therefore, coinciding in time with the biopsychosocial model of health, systems theory was also influential in shaping an understanding of health. Systems theory was used to conceptualize individuals as consisting of layers of systems, such as cells, organs, physiological systems and, at a broader level, biological and psychological systems as well as existing within external systems such as the broader social, sociocultural systems in which the person lived. In this theory, people were conceptualized as open systems, in which they received input from the external environment (external systems) and were also able to act upon it (the mutual influence of different systems, both internal and external).

The occupational therapy models of the 1990s were particularly influenced by biopsychosocial and systems understandings of humans, usually making explicit the performance components (based on the impairment focus of the biomedical model of health) presented in earlier models along with attention to subjective experience and psychological concerns such as identity. The concept of stress was also made explicit as acknowledgement increased of the importance to health of people's sociocultural environment. In addition, because the broader systems surrounding the individual were attended to, the occupational therapy models at this time also identified different aspects of the environment, both physical and social, with which the individual interacted.

A common criticism of the biopsychosocial model of health is that, while it conceptualizes the individual as influenced by his or her broader context, it remains focused on the individual. Increasingly, current Western concepts of health are interested in the factors that affect the health of populations, rather than viewing health primarily as an individual concern. In addition, indigenous and Eastern ways of thinking and acting are becoming more available to the Western world, and the collective nature of people's lives is becoming more overtly acknowledged. Consequently, Western health care appears to be increasingly influenced by a third model, a socioecological model of health.

A socioecological model of health attends to the broader patterns of health distribution in a society. It is concerned with the fact that "some people have poorer health than others do and, more importantly, that certain groups of people have poorer health than others" (Reidpath, 2004, p. 9). Consequently, it conceptualizes health as determined by a much greater range of factors than biological abnormality or factors relating specifically to an individual. A determinant of health is defined as "a factor or characteristic that brings about a change in health, either for the better or for the worse" (Reidpath, p. 9). Determinants of health include a diverse range of factors such as exercise, the quality of the water supply, exposure to the sun, and the conditions in which people work and live. They can be categorized as social, environmental, biological and genetic. Because the way a society is structured can advantage or disadvantage different groups (e.g. statistically the wealthiest are the healthiest), a socioecological model of health is concerned with health inequality (the unequal distribution of health, i.e. why some groups in society are healthier than others) and equity of access to health services and other factors that are protective of health (e.g. safe working conditions).

To date, occupational therapy appears to have been primarily characterized by a biopsychosocial perspective. This is evident in the individual focus of many occupational therapy models. However, this situation might currently be changing. Many of the current versions of models explicitly state that clients can be populations and groups rather than just individuals. In addition, in closer alignment with a socioecological view, the Canadian Model of Occupational Performance and Engagement (CMOP-E) makes explicit the issue of equity regarding health and participation, through its concern for a just society, and includes advocacy (and power sharing) as a key enablement skill.

It may be, as we progress further into the twenty-first century and broader views become more widely accepted within health models, that occupational therapy theory and practice pursues more explicitly this direction away from an individual focus. The practice of occupational therapy might change in response to changes in the broader societies in which occupational therapists work. For example, Western countries might continue to broaden their concepts of health and well-being and confront pressing issues such as the disadvantages and poorer health often seen in indigenous populations. Similarly, the philosophies and world views of people in non-Western countries might increasingly influence occupational therapy theory and practice (in both Western and non-Western countries).

While the influence of the three models of health is evident within the occupational therapy models presented in this book, there are three themes that also run through the way occupational therapy has organized its concepts over time. First, during the 1970s, authors primarily aimed to make explicit the fundamental beliefs of occupational therapy. At this time, these thinking frameworks were generally not called models and focused on developing a conceptual system that integrated major ideas about interventions for particular population groups.

Second, from the mid and late 1980s, the focus became the explication of ways of organizing information into schemes that generally were referred to as models. The occupational performance models published by the American and Canadian occupational therapy associations were primarily influenced by a biomedical understanding of health. Other models used the language of systems theory. For example, the Model of Human Occupation (MOHO), published as its first edition in 1985, and the person-environment-performance model published in 1991 by Christiansen and Baum, both made explicit their basis in open systems theory. Table I.2 provides an overview of the models reviewed in this book, their respective publication years and the models of health with which they are associated.

The third theme evident within contemporary models is the language of occupation. While occupation (human action) is widely accepted as the core of occupational therapy practice, occupational therapy models vary as to whether occupation is presented as a discrete entity within the model or is more like the largely invisible lens through which person and environment are viewed. Throughout this book, we will use the analogy of looking out a window to refer to the place of occupation in the various models. Windows are transparent so that you can look through them to something else. At times, your focus might be on what you can see through the window and you might be largely unaware of the window itself. At other times, your attention might include awareness of the way the window frames and shapes what you see through it (Figure I.1).

Using this metaphor, some of the earlier occupational therapy models were structured as if one was looking through the window of occupation at the person and environment. In these models, the main focus is on the interaction between person and environment and occupation appears to be the accepted purpose of the model but not necessarily a component of the model. In other models, it is as if the person doing the looking has taken a step back and described the process of looking out the window, where the window itself is included in the description of what can be seen. Therefore, the more recent models, and editions of older models, tend to include occupation as a discrete component within the model (with the exception of CMOP-E). A mutually influencing interaction between person, environment and occupation is presented, rather than focusing on the interaction between person and environment in order to understand occupation.

Occupational therapy models also vary in their conceptualization of the relationship between occupation and human health and well-being. Some models are based on the assumption that occupation is the *vehicle* through

USING OCCUPATIONAL THERAPY MODELS IN PRACTICE

| Table 1.2 | Occupational therapy models covered in this book | |
|---|---|---|
| **Model** | **Publication year/s** | **Model of health** |
| Occupational Performance Model (OPM) (Pedretti) | 1981, 1985, 1990, 1996, 2001 | Primarily biomedical |
| Occupational Performance Model (Australia) (OPMA) (Chapparo & Ranka) | 1997 | Biopsychosocial |
| Occupational Adaptation (OA) (Schkade & Schultz) | 1992, 1997, 2001, 2003, 2009 | Biopsychosocial |
| Person Environment Occupation Performance (PEOP) (Christiansen & Baum) | 1991, 1997, 2005 | Biopsychosocial |
| Person Environment Occupation (PEO) (Law et al.) | 1996 | Primarily biopsychosocial (objective and subjective aspects of person important & the interconnectedness associated with systems theory), with some socioecological (event is the unit of focus rather than individual, but does not focus on patterns of health distribution) |
| Ecology of Human Performance (EHP) (Dunn, Brown & McQuigan) | 1994 | Socioecological and biopsychosocial (context is the lens through which occupational performance is viewed) |
| Canadian Model of Occupational Performance (CMOP) (CAOT) and Canadian Model of Occupational Performance & Engagement (CMOP-E) (Townsend & Polatajko) | 1997, 2002, 2007 | Biopsychosocial with the 2007 edition tending to encompass socioecological issues as well (such as social justice) |
| Model of Human Occupation (MOHO) (Kielhofner) | 1985, 1995, 2002, 2008 | Biopsychosocial |
| Kawa model (Iwama) | 2006 | Doesn't conform to the major Western models of health (Western practitioners have to be careful that they don't interpret it from a biopsychosocial perspective). Probably aligns most closely with socioecological |

which humans influence their environment. This approach seems to flow from the early occupational therapy proposition that obtaining mastery over the environment is central to good health and well-being. In occupational therapy, the ability of the person to obtain mastery over his or her surroundings has been proposed to enhance survival (Clark, 1997; Reed & Sanderson, 1999; Wilcock, 1993), facilitate growth and development (Gilfoyle et al., 1981;

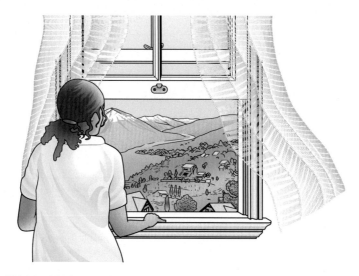

FIG 1.1    Window metaphor — picture of a person looking through a window.

Nelson, 1988) and self-actualization (Baum & Christiansen, 1997) and contribute to improved quality of life (Goldberg et al., 2002). The importance of
obtaining mastery over the environment shaped the early profession.

In contrast, some models do not separate the person and environment in
the same way and, therefore, do not conceptualize occupation as a vehicle for
mastery over the environment. For example, the ecological models emphasize
the interconnectedness of person and environment and stress that they should
not be conceptualized as separate entities. Similarly, the concept of the decentralized self in the Kawa model means that obtaining mastery over something
that is essentially part of the self makes little sense.

The conceptualization of person and environment as distinct entities and
occupation as the medium through which one acts upon the other is not an
assumption evident in all occupational therapy models. While the concept
of mastery over the environment was foundational to the profession of occupational therapy, it appears that this concept, which could have become an
unspoken assumption, might require discussion and clarification in the future.

## USING MODELS IN PRACTICE

Exploring models is one way to develop an understanding of the concepts
upon which the profession of occupational therapy is based. However, for
that to be a worthwhile endeavour, the process should lead to an enhanced
understanding that can facilitate the practice of occupational therapy.
Therefore, this book is really about using models in practice rather than
understanding them as an end in themselves. What models essentially do
is provide an organizing framework with which to think about practice in
a systematic way, and to provide a discourse with which to discuss practice
with others. Professional practice is recognized as a complex and messy
process. Without some process for making sense of the complicated situations

in which therapists find themselves, professional practice can become haphazard and dependent upon the individual occupational therapist.

Professions are communities with which their members identify while they practice in different settings with a variety of clients. Lave and Wenger (1991) used the term "communities of practice" (p. 29) to refer to the communities to which individuals belong and within which they engage in learning in a specific context. These communities of practice represent and express the shared understandings that characterize a particular profession and distinguish it from other professional groups. Conceptual frameworks help individual occupational therapists to organize their work in line with the shared understandings of their profession. In phenomenological terms, these shared understandings are referred to as professional "habits of mind" (Toombs, 1992). This concept emphasizes that professions cannot simply be distinguished by their processes, procedures and tools, but that each brings particular and habitual perspectives with which to understand and interpret phenomena. The concept of habit expresses that there is something automatic about this perspective in that habits enable people to act without necessarily requiring conscious effort. The term *habit of mind* creates the sense that professionals, through their training, see the world through a professional lens of which they might no longer be conscious.

Models of practice provide a language to help individual occupational therapists articulate to others the perspective that is unique to their profession. They make explicit the concepts upon which the profession is based and how concepts are grouped or organized together. Thus, they are important for strengthening the professional identities of occupational therapists by providing a language with which to express to others their habitual ways of making sense of the world and the value of their professional perspective for their clients.

## OVERVIEW OF THE BOOK

In order to facilitate the use of models in practice, this book aims to provide an overview of a range of different occupational therapy models, placed within the conceptual context of practice. As a fieldguide, it aims to provide a resource for occupational therapists and occupational therapy students whilst engaged in professional practice. Chapters 1 and 2 provide the context within which to think about the use of models in practice. Chapter 1 discusses the concepts of theory and practice and their relationship. It presents theory as a way of thinking that arises from and aims to make sense of practice. It also discusses the different types and sources of knowledge that occupational therapists might use in practice. Chapter 2 uses the framework of professional reasoning to explore how models can be used to guide what occupational therapists 'see' in their practice and how they think about it. It presents the Model of Context-specific Professional Reasoning (MCPR) to assist occupational therapists to consider the various contexts that affect their work. Chapters 3 to 7 specifically overview a selection of occupational therapy models. For each model, an overview of its purpose and structure is provided, along with a diagrammatic representation of the model, and then the development of the model is discussed. To facilitate its use in practice, a memory aide is provided to guide the clinician when using the model during practice. In addition, the major works relating to each model and a case illustration are provided. To help readers to see some of the similarities in various models, some are grouped within one chapter. Chapter 3 focuses on individual occupational performance and adaptation and includes occupational performance models from the United States of America and Australia and the Occupational Adaptation model. Chapter 4 includes models that attend in to person, environment and occupation, rather than focusing especially on the individual. Three models are presented in separate chapters as their organization and/or emphasis differs from some of the other models. Chapter 5 presents the Canadian Model of Occupational Performance and Engagement (CMOP-E), Chapter 6 the Model of Human Occupation (MOHO) and Chapter 7 the Kawa model. Finally, Chapter 8 provides a discussion of the trends in occupational therapy that are evident within the models reviewed in this book.

## REFERENCES

Baum, C., Christiansen, C., 1997. The occupational therapy context: Philosophy – principles – practice. In: Christiansen, C., Baum, C. (Eds.), Occupational therapy: Enabling function and well-being, second ed.. Slack, Thorofare, NJ, pp. 26–45.

Clark, F., 1997. Reflections on the human as an occupational being: Biological need, tempo and temporality. J. Occup. Sci. Aust. 4 (3), 86–92.

Engel, G.L., 1977. The need for a new medical model: a challenge for biomedicine. Science 196: 129–136.

Gilfoyle, E.M., Grady, A.P., Moore, J.C., 1981. Children adapt. Slack, Thorofare, NJ.

Goldberg, B., Brintnell, E., Goldberg, J., 2002. The relationship between engagement in meaningful activities and quality of life in persons disabled by mental illness. Occup. Ther. Mental Health 18, 17–44.

Good, B., DelVecchio Good, M.J., 1980. The meaning of symptoms: A cultural hermeneutic model for clinical practice. In: Eisenberg, I., Kleinman, A. (Eds.), The relevance of social science for medicine. Reidel, Norwell, MA, pp. 165–196.

Kielhofner, G., 2009. Conceptual foundations of occupational therapy, fourth ed. F.A. Davis, Philadelphia, PA.

Lave, J., Wenger, E., 1991. Situated learning: legitimate peripheral participation. Cambridge University Press, New York.

Nelson, D., 1988. Occupation: Form and performance. Am. J. Occup. Ther. 42 (10), 633–641.

Reed, K., 2005. An annotated history of the concepts used in occupational therapy, In: Christiansen, C.H., Baum, C.M., Bass-Haugen, J. (Eds.), Occupational therapy: Performance, participation, and well-being, third ed. Slack, Thorofare, NJ, pp. 567–626.

Reed, K.L., Sanderson, S.N., 1999. Concepts of occupational therapy, fourth ed. Williams & Wilkins, Baltimore, MD.

Reidpath, D., 2004. Social determinants of health. In: Keleher, H., Murphy, B. (Eds.), Understanding health: a determinants approach. Oxford University Press, Melbourne, VIC, pp. 9–22.

Taylor, S., Field, D., 2003. Approaches to health and health care. In: Taylor, S., Field, D. (Eds.), Sociology of health and health care. Blackwell, Oxford, pp. 21–42.

Toombs, S.K., 1992. The meaning of illness: a phenomenological account of the different perspectives of physicians and patient. Kluwer Academic Publishers, Dordrecht; Boston.

Whiteford, G., Townsend, E., Hocking, C., 2000. Reflections on a renaissance of occupation. Can. J. Occup. Ther. 67 (1), 61–69.

Wilcock, A., 1993. A theory of the human need for occupation. J. Occup. Sci. Aust. 1 (1), 17–24.

# Theory and practice

In this book, and beginning with this chapter, we draw upon the idea that different ways of knowing are required for practice. Rather than taking the perspective that theory precedes and is applied to practice, we use practice as our starting point and ask how theory can *serve* practice.

## WHAT ARE THEORY AND PRACTICE AND WHY DO THEY MATTER?

In occupational therapy, theory has been defined as a set of connected ideas or concepts that can be used to guide or form the basis for action (Crepeau et al., 2009; Melton et al., 2009). If a given theory is good, it can be used to explain phenomena as well as predict the likely outcomes of changes to those phenomena. Because they are made explicit, theories can be scrutinized and tested (Melton et al., 2009).

Theories form part of a profession's body of knowledge. Higgs et al. (2001) explained that, without a theoretical base, practice would be akin to guesswork. While experienced occupational therapists often have difficulty explaining the theoretical bases for their practice, the fact that they make well-reasoned and effective decisions after gaining very little information (Mattingly & Fleming, 1994) suggests that they are not engaged in 'guesswork' but are combining the information obtained with their body of knowledge. As Melton et al. (2009) explained, disciplines develop

13

© 2011 Elsevier Ltd.
DOI: 10.1016/B978-0-7234-3494-8.00001-2

"a specialized knowledge base, important concepts, models and theories to help busy practitioners make rapid but well-informed decisions about their practice" (p. 12). In occupational therapy, Crepeau et al. (2009) stated that its theoretical knowledge base "concerns occupation, how occupation influences health and well-being, and how occupation can be used therapeutically to enable people to engage in those occupations they value most" (p. 429).

Melton et al. (2009) proposed that providing a "framework of conceptual ideas" serves purposes such as the following:

- "having a structure upon which to locate thinking, reasoning and the construction of practice-based decisions;
- guidance in selecting research evidence, assessments and interventions that most appropriately link with the essence of occupational therapy practice;
- having a language with which to articulate the occupational needs of the client;
- having resources with which to build professional know-how into expertise; and
- better matching of service user needs and aspirations with the provision of theory" (p. 12).

## PRACTICE IS MORE THAN THEORY

While theory appears to be essential for practice, it is rarely considered to be sufficient for practice. The practice of occupational therapy refers to what occupational therapists do in their professional roles. It is a process that requires decision-making about action and can be thought of as *reasoned action* (Carr, 1995). Sometimes practice is conceptualized as the application of theory, but Mattingly and Fleming (1994) proposed that practice is much more than this because it requires a different type of reasoning.

Both theory and practice are important for the work of professionals. However, they are not the same. Higgs et al. (2001) distinguished between knowing *that* and knowing *how*. Theory can be thought of as knowing *that*. By making explicit what a particular profession knows about, theory is essential to both the organization and sharing of the profession's knowledge base in its area of concern. On the other hand, practice is more aligned with knowing *how*. It requires both skills, in particular aspects of the profession's work and the ability to choose action (or non-action) wisely.

## DIFFERENT TYPES OF KNOWLEDGE

In discussing the difference between theory and practice, some authors (e.g. Higgs et al. 2001; Mattingly & Fleming, 1994) refer back to the ancient philosophies of Plato and Aristotle. While both philosophers agreed that there are different types of knowledge, Plato argued for the superiority of the type of knowledge associated with mathematics. This kind of knowledge was called *episteme* and gives rise to the term epistemology. This type of knowledge is: (a) propositional, that is, it comprises a set of assertions or propositions that can be explained, studied and transmitted in words and often includes assertions of truth; (b) generalized, aiming to state universal principles; and (c) purely intellectual (rather than emotional). It is generally associated with a scientific way of thinking and is the type of knowledge that the word theory usually conjures.

The type of knowledge that is often associated with practice is *phronesis* or practical wisdom. As Kessels and Korthagen (1996) explained, "this is an essentially different type of knowledge, not concerned with scientific theories, but with the understanding of specific concrete cases and complex or ambiguous situations" (p. 19). This type of knowledge is situated in and relevant to particular times and places. As Aristotle stated, while phronesis can involve general principles, "It must take into account particular facts as well, since it is concerned with practical activities, which always deal with particular things" (Aristotle, 1975, p. 1141). Practice requires more than just knowing information and is often distinguished by the need to act in a particular situation (even if it is only to make decisions, a form of action). Understanding a situation is dependent on experience, which allows the practitioner to see patterns and similarities (upon which to base practice 'rules') in a series of particular instances. As Kessels and Korthagen explained, "particulars only become familiar with experience, with a long process of perceiving, assessing situations, judging, choosing courses of action, and being confronted with their consequences" (p. 20).

Often, theories are conceptualized as being 'applied' to practice, the implication being that theory somehow precedes (and is possibly superior to) practice. Certainly, most occupational therapy courses in Western countries are structured with theoretical concepts taught first and more extensive professional practice experiences occurring later. An extensive knowledge of theory – generally conceptualized as generalized, propositional knowledge – is consistent with society's expectation of professionals as 'experts'. Mattingly and Fleming (1994) explained that, in the health professions, the reasoning required has generally been conceptualized as "applied natural science" in which "reasoning is presumed to involve recognizing particular instances of behaviour in terms of general laws that regulate the relationship between cause and a resultant state of affairs" and that "practice is considered the application of empirically tested abstract knowledge (theories) and generalizable factual knowledge" (p. 317).

Higgs et al. (2001) identified three forms of knowledge that professionals use. The first of these, *propositional knowledge*, is the type of knowledge that is most associated with professions and aligns most closely with the concept of episteme. It is also known as theory or scientific knowledge. As Higgs et al. explained:

*Propositional knowledge is formal and explicit, and is expressed in propositional statements. Relationships between concepts or cause and effect, for example, are set out. This form of knowledge is derived through research and/or scholarship. Claims about the generalizability or transferability of research knowledge to settings other than that in which the investigation was carried out are made. (p. 5)*

Propositional knowledge is the type of knowledge that underpins the concept of the 'expert'. It forms an important part of the professional knowledge base, which is often associated with broad principles that can be generalized to a range of different settings. The particularity of various knowledge bases helps to distinguish one profession from another.

The second type of knowledge identified was *professional craft knowledge*. This type of knowledge is based on experience in practice and relates to knowing how to do something. It includes the skills required to practice; knowing from experience about particular client groups, the types of problems that they might face and the kinds of interventions that are often useful to them; and knowledge about the particular client with whom the professional is working at the time. As Higgs et al. stated, "Professional craft knowledge can be expressed in propositional statements, but here no attempt is made to generalize beyond the individual's or a group of colleagues' own practice" (p. 5). Thus, professional craft knowledge is often highly context-specific, rather than generalized (or necessarily generalizable) like propositional knowledge. As a practical form of knowledge, it aligns most closely with *phronesis*.

The third type of knowledge is *personal knowledge*. This includes the professional's knowledge of him- or herself as a person and in relation to others. It is built up over the course of a person's life and can relate to the social mores that the individual professional has experienced (and internalized or rejected), his or her world view, and any knowledge of him- or herself as a person that may have been developed through reflection and experience.

While theoretical knowledge can be conceptualized as propositional knowledge, the other two types of knowledge are primarily examples of 'non-propositional' knowledge (Higgs et al., 2001, p. 5). The distinction between propositional and non-propositional knowledge relates, respectively, to the difference between *knowing that* and *knowing how* (Polanyi, 1958; Ryle, 1949) mentioned earlier. It also aligns with the distinction Mattingly and Fleming (1994) made between theoretical and practical reasoning. In contrast to propositional knowledge, which exists in the public sphere through wide dissemination, non-propositional knowledge is often "tacit and embedded" (Higgs et al., p. 5), that is, not necessarily put into words or easy to explain but embedded in the action of practice.

Aligning with the concept of propositional and non-propositional knowledge being important aspects of practice, Crepeau et al. (2009) distinguished between formal and personal theories. Formal theories are those that are "publicly articulated, published and validated to varying degrees by scientific study" (p. 429). Personal theories are those beliefs held by individuals. They are formed through the individual's experiences and perspectives formed from observations and exposure to ideas and beliefs. They are not made widely available and, therefore, are less likely to have been publicly scrutinized and debated.

## IMPLICATIONS OF DIFFERENT TYPES OF KNOWLEDGE

The distinction between personal and formal theories is important to consider in relation to the current emphasis in health on evidence-based practice (EBP). The desire to provide quality and cost-effective services that have a positive impact of outcomes for clients and patients is widely shared by a range of stakeholder groups including clients, health professionals, managers of services and funding bodies (Turpin & Higgs, 2010). However, there is a lack of consensus as to how to achieve these outcomes. In its approach to achieving these outcomes, the EBP movement generally values formal theories over personal theories. It promotes the use of knowledge that has been generated and tested using rigorous research methods such as randomized controlled trials and their systematic reviews. The emphasis on research findings that are generalizable to situations other than those in which the results were generated aims to overcome the limitations in reasoning that have been noted in professionals. As Duncan (2006) explained, "it is known that professionals' individual perspectives are highly vulnerable to a range of biases and heuristics when making clinical judgements" (p. 60).

A problem facing practitioners is that, if they only rely on their own experiences of phenomena in the local context, they are likely to make their decisions based on a reasonably narrow range of choices. These are often influenced by factors other than effectiveness of interventions (the focus of EBP). An example includes the difference between a practitioner's extensive knowledge of the services they can provide and their relative lack of knowledge of the interventions that another professional or service could provide (and the research outlining the effectiveness or otherwise of these interventions).

On the other hand, the advantage of personal theories is that they are based on experience within the particular practice context and knowledge of, and the capacity to respond to, individual variations in client preferences and needs. Sackett (2000) defined evidence-based medicine (upon which EBP in occupational therapy is based) as "the integration of best research evidence with clinical expertise and patient values" (p. 1). This definition suggests that both formal and personal theories may be constitutive of EBP.

There is much discussion about theory and practice in professional disciplines. In these discussions, frequent reference is made to a 'gap' between theory and practice. Examples from a range of disciplines include education (Kessels & Korthagen, 1996), nursing (Rolfe, 1998), physiotherapy (Rothstein, 2004), and occupational therapy (Melton et al., 2009). The concept of the theory–practice gap provides a way of articulating the problem inherent within professional practice of having to integrate different types of knowledge from different sources when making decisions about professional action. While definitions of evidence-based practice, such as the one by Sackett (2000) quoted before, refer to the integration of different types of information, little has been done to investigate the process of integration.

Valuing, and therefore having to combine, different types of knowledge in practice is particularly powerful within occupational therapy. The equal valuing of both propositional and non-propositional knowledge has been expressed in occupational therapy through concepts such as *art and science* and the 'two-body practice' (Mattingly & Fleming, 1994). In addition, through its focus on occupation as both a means to facilitate occupational performance and participation and an end in itself, the practice of occupational therapy requires both theory about occupation and practical guidance on how to use occupation to achieve these aims (theory and practice or episteme and phronesis).

In this section, a range of different terminology is reviewed in relation to the occupational therapy discourse about theory and practice. A historical approach to understanding this terminology has been taken, as the way occupational therapy has used terminology relating to theory and practice appears to have changed over time. The ways that a variety of authors have categorized theory are discussed.

There are historical differences in the way terms have been used to describe the various levels of theory referred to in occupational therapy. Mosey, an important writer about occupational therapy theory in the 1970s, 80s and early 90s, distinguished between a profession's "fundamental body of knowledge" (p. 49) and its "applied body of knowledge" (p. 69). She stated that, "a profession's fundamental body of knowledge is a compilation of all the information a profession recognises as basic to, and supportive of, its applied body of knowledge and practice. The information is typically a combination of philosophical and scientific knowledge drawn from a variety of sources. It may also include some practical knowledge" (p. 49). Mosey identified five categories of knowledge within a profession's fundamental body of knowledge. These were philosophical assumptions (basic beliefs), an ethical code, theoretical foundations ("theories and empirical data that serve as a scientific basis for practice" [p. 63]), a domain of concern and legitimate tools.

Mosey (1992) explained that a profession also requires an applied body of knowledge, which is compatible with the fundamental body of knowledge, because the latter "is not meant to be used directly" (p. 69). She defined an applied body of knowledge as "a collection of information formulated so that it serves as the basis for day-to-day problem identification and resolution with clients" and proposed that it included a profession's "sets of guidelines for practice" (p. 69). She commented that, while a range of different terms might be used for these guidelines, including terms like practice theory, model of practice and ground rules, all of these terms refer to "the transformation of theoretical knowledge into a form that allow[s] it to be used in practice" (p. 73).

Mosey (1992) provided examples of two sets of guidelines for practice; diagnostic categories in medicine and frames of reference in occupational therapy. She explained that a frame of reference includes: (a) its theoretical base that "defines and describes the nature of the area of human experience to which the frame of reference is addressed" (p. 85); (b) the relevant function–dysfunction continua which define the way that problem areas are understood and how they are resolved; (c) the behaviours and physical signs that indicate function and dysfunction; and (d) the postulates (statements or precepts) outlining the actions that are expected to lead to change (usually to enhance function – in whatever way that is conceptualized in the frame of reference).

Mosey (1992) saw frames of reference as relevant to a particular profession. For example, she stated, "it should be remembered that a frame of reference is only one type of *sets of guidelines* for practice. Frames of reference are not suitable for medicine, just as diagnostic categories are not suitable for occupational therapy. Each profession, then, has a type of *sets of guidelines* to meet its own particular practice needs" (p. 87).

In contrast to Mosey's definition, some current authors use the term *frame of reference* to refer to bodies of knowledge that occupational therapists use that are *not* specific to occupational therapy. Crepeau et al. (2009) stated that "frames of reference guide practice by delineating the beliefs, assumptions, definitions, and concepts within a specific area of practice". An example of this categorization includes theoretical frameworks such as developmental, cognitive-behavioural, psychodynamic and biomechanical theoretical frameworks (Duncan, 2006; Reel & Feaver, 2006). Categorizing frames of reference as those approaches that guide practice in a specific area means that specific perspectives can be included regardless of whether they are specific to occupational therapy or not. Consequently, the examples of frames of reference provided by a number of authors include approaches that are broader than occupational therapy such as motor control, self-advocacy and rehabilitation as well as frameworks that are specific to occupational therapy practice, such as the AOTA Practice Guidelines.

Writing to a broader interdisciplinary audience, Reel and Feaver (2006) listed eight terms that are often used to discuss theory and practice in rehabilitation. These were frames of reference, domains, treatment approaches, paradigms, perspectives, models, philosophies and techniques. In organizing this list they first considered philosophy to be a broader concept and cited Craig's (1983 in Reel & Feaver, 2006) definition as follows: "A philosophy is a creed, a set of beliefs to live by; it provides a purpose encompassing and overriding the minor and trivial concerns of the everyday, or if not, it communicates a state of mind from within which the ultimate purposelessness of life becomes bearable" (p. 53). They proposed that the various disciplines working in rehabilitation have their own philosophies but also have shared philosophies. Examples of the latter were healthcare ethics, client-centred practice and a developmental/lifelong context. They defined professional philosophy as "the system of beliefs and values unique to each profession, which provides its members with a sense of identity and exerts control over theory and practice. It helps locate the domains of concern for that profession – irrespective of the particular practice context" (p. 53). They defined frames of reference as "clusters of theories selected or developed by different professionals out of the need to support the philosophical beliefs that are the core of the profession" and stated that "Frames of reference give principles on which to base specific intervention. Frames of reference are aimed at specific problems and professionals choose from a number of appropriate frames of reference." (p. 55). In comparing philosophy and frames of reference, they suggested that philosophies (and paradigms) represented a 'softer' type of knowledge and that frames of reference are based on the 'harder' sciences (p. 56).

The way terms are used in occupational therapy varies widely and is dependent on the system each author uses for classifying different levels of theory. Generally, the term Frame of Reference is favoured for theoretical systems that are not specifically limited to the profession of occupational therapy. This term often appears to be used interchangeably with terms such as treatment or intervention approaches because they often provide a level of detail that enables their direct use in practice. Theoretical frameworks that deal with occupation are considered to be specific to the profession of occupational therapy and are generally referred to as conceptual models of practice.

In occupational therapy, Cole and Tufano (2008) identified three levels of theory. These were paradigm, occupation-based models and frames of reference. They used the term paradigm to "incorporate some of what Mosey called our fundamental body of knowledge" (p. 57), and included the philosophical basis for occupational therapy, its values and ethics, and "three concepts most basic to practice in the OT profession: occupation, purposeful activity, and function" (p. 57). They drew upon the AOTA Occupational Therapy Practice Framework, proposing that it creates a classification system "for OT knowledge that is consistent with our paradigm" (p. 59). Their second level was occupation-based models. They explained that these have also been referred to as overarching frames of reference, conceptual models and occupation-based frameworks. They stated that, "in OT, occupation-based models help explain the relationships among the person, the environment, and occupational performance, forming the foundation for the profession's focus on occupation" (p. 57). Included in this level are Occupational Behaviour, Model of Human Occupation, Occupational Adaptation, Ecology of Human Performance, and Person-Environment-Occupational-Performance Model. Their third level, called frames of reference, referred to practice guidelines in specific domains. This level included frameworks such as Applied Behavioural Frames, Cognitive Behavioural Frames, Biomechanical and Rehabilitative Frames, Allen's Cognitive Levels Frame and a range of other 'frames'.

Kielhofner (2009) presented knowledge relevant to occupational therapy as three concentric circles with paradigm in the middle of the circle, conceptual practice models as the next layer and related knowledge as the outer layer. Paradigm refers to the shared or common vision of the discipline and includes core constructs, a focal viewpoint and values. Kielhofner proposed that the paradigm helps to unify the profession and define its nature and purpose. Conceptual practice models provide the details that guide occupational therapists in their practice and he contended that they consist of theory, practice resources and a research and evidence base. In contrast to the previous two layers, related knowledge comprises knowledge and skills that are not unique to occupational therapy. He provided examples such as knowledge of medical diagnoses and disease processes and cognitive and behavioural concepts and skills from psychology.

Duncan's (2006) categorization of levels of theory is consistent with that of Kielhofner (1997, 2009). He used three theoretical categories to structure his presentation of occupational therapy frameworks. These were: (a) paradigm, which was defined as "the shared consensus regarding the most fundamental beliefs of the profession"; (b) frame of reference, which he conceptualized as a theoretical framework that was developed outside of the profession but can be applicable to occupational therapy (similar to Kielhofner's related knowledge); and (c) conceptual models of practice, which are occupation-based and were developed specifically to explain occupational therapy practice and processes. Examples of conceptual models of practice provided were MOHO, CMOP, the Functional Information-processing model, Activities Therapy: a recapitulation of ontogenesis and the Kawa model. The frames of reference provided were the client-centred frame of reference, the cognitive-behavioural frame of reference, the psychodynamic frame of reference, the biomechanical frame of reference, and approaches to motor control and cognitive-perceptual function.

In this book, we use the term models of practice (often abbreviated to models) to refer to occupational therapy frameworks that relate to practice. We have not included theoretical or philosophical frameworks or specific frames of reference that exist to guide practice in a specific area.

## PRACTICE AS A STARTING POINT: MODELS SERVING OCCUPATIONAL THERAPY PRACTICE

In this book, we draw upon the idea that different ways of knowing are required for practice. Rather than taking the perspective that theory precedes and is applied to practice, we use practice as our starting point and ask how theory can *serve* practice. Emphasizing the difference between 'serving' and 'applying to' allows us to address the taken-for-granted assumption in Western society that theoretical knowledge has a higher intrinsic value than practical wisdom. As this book is about practice, and aims to provide a useful resource for practitioners, we centre our attention firmly on practice and how theory can be used in practice. As Kielhofner (1995) stated, "Theory can never tell therapists, in advance, exactly what should be done in the context of therapy. But, if therapists understand a theory, it will help them figure out what to do at the time. Practice requires therapists to imagine how persons might find their ways out of states of dysfunction and achieve better lives. Theory which supports such therapeutic imagining cannot offer a simple plan or recipe. Rather, it must sharpen and deepen the quality of a therapist's thinking." (p. 1).

As the purpose of this book is to provide resources to assist occupational therapists in practice, only those conceptual frameworks that are specific to occupational therapy are included. As discussed earlier, these are often referred to as conceptual models of practice as their purpose is to present a system of ideas that can be used to guide practice. Thus, they are developed to link theory and practice together.

Occupational therapy appears to be a practice in which the development of models of practice has been important. The nature of occupational therapy theory and practice may have contributed to the proliferation of models of practice in two ways. First, occupational therapy focuses on occupational engagement and participation in everyday life. Therefore, the practice of occupational therapy can appear from outside the profession like 'common sense' because it centres on ordinary doing. However, occupational therapy practice could better be described as *uncommon sense* because occupational therapists provide unique ways of looking at various aspects of ordinary doing. They use this unique perspective to enable people who face barriers to occupational performance to participate fully in their daily lives and societies. However, this uncommon sense needs to be articulated clearly to others who might only be able to see the outcomes that relate to people doing ordinary things. It is likely that making explicit occupational therapy's unique perspective serves to assist people to see the value of the contribution that occupational therapy can make to people's lives and to see that it is not simply common sense. Without such explicitness, the value of occupational therapy could go unnoticed because engagement in occupation and participation in society are taken for granted and, therefore, often invisible until disrupted. Occupational therapy models of practice are one way that the practice makes its uniqueness overt and explicit.

## 1

The second reason why models of practice could have become prolific in occupational therapy is because of its basis in pragmatism, a discipline of philosophy. Pragmatism emphasizes the connection between theory and practice (Encarta, 2009), that is, between thought and action. This connection appears to operate at two levels within occupational therapy. First, occupational therapists are concerned about both what people do and how they think about those actions. This concern is usually articulated through the concept of meaningful occupation. That is, occupational therapists attend to what people *think* about the things they do, as well as about what and how they do them. The second way that the connection between thought and action is evident in occupational therapy is in the way that occupational therapists work. Mattingly and Fleming (1994) emphasized that *thinking in action* is central to occupational therapists' reasoning. Thus, the distinction that is often made between theory and practice might not be relevant to the way occupational therapists work. While it is accepted that they need to have a firm base of knowledge upon which to base their practice, occupational therapists quickly turn their knowledge (whether pre-existing generalized knowledge or specific knowledge about clients and their particular circumstances) into action. They also acquire new knowledge through action. Models of practice aim to assist therapists by providing a conceptual framework for thinking about, planning and interpreting action (both theirs and that of their clients). While other levels of theory might aim to address issues such as philosophy, models of practice aim to link theory and practice together.

## WAYS MODELS OF PRACTICE SERVE PRACTICE

Models of practice aim to guide practice by providing a basis for decision-making. They are specific to occupational therapy and encapsulate the values and beliefs of the profession. Because occupation is the core of occupational therapy, they all deal with occupation in a central way. Models of practice *serve* practice in a variety of ways.

First, models of practice make the profession's assumptions about humans and occupation explicit. In explaining the relevant concepts and their relationships, each model makes explicit the assumptions upon which it is based. For the model to be accepted as appropriate to occupational therapy, it has to be based on the assumptions of the profession. While occupational therapists will have to initially put time and energy into understanding a particular model, once they are familiar with it, the structure of the model can usually be used to guide practice. That is, the assumptions underpinning the model become internalized and the person using it does not need to constantly refer to its assumptions each time they use it. Therefore, models of practice essentially provide a 'short-cut' for guiding professional reasoning. By using the model properly, professionals can have confidence they are being faithful to the assumptions of the profession.

Second, models of practice help to define the scope of practice. They have embedded within them assumptions about the domain of concern of occupational therapy. They shape the way that professionals 'see' their practice and they provide guidance about what falls within the scope of practice and what does not. They provide a focus for the occupational therapist and define the parameters of factors and information that should be included in the planning of assessment and intervention. Some models provide specific guidance through the development of assessments that deal specifically with the model's concepts. Occupational therapists are guided to pay particular attention to those things that are within the scope of their practice and to know when other professionals or services might be best dealing with other things.

Third, models of practice can enhance professionalism and accountability. Three criteria form the basis for claims of professional status. These are: (1) an independent body of knowledge and expertise, with a university degree as a minimum standard of education; (2) recognition of professional status at a state (government) level; and (3) self-regulation (autonomy) through ethical decision-making guided by a code of ethics (Williams, 2005). In making explicit the theoretical assumptions of the profession upon which they are based, models of practice contribute to this demonstration of an independent body of knowledge.

Higgs et al. (2001) stressed the importance of professional accountability and of reviewing critically their professional knowledge base and making it publically available. Models of practice are a way that the profession makes explicit its knowledge base and can contribute to the critical review of that knowledge base. The historical approach that we have taken in this book emphasizes this function of models by discussing the reasons for the model's development and any perceived gap in the profession's discourse or emphasis that the model aimed to fill.

Fourth, models of practice assist occupational therapists to be systematic and comprehensive in their collection of information. In general, models aim to guide occupational therapists to develop a holistic understanding of their clients. Each aims to set out a holistic theoretical framework (as the authors see it at the time of the model's development or revision), which can be used to assist occupational therapists to avoid some of the problems inherent in human reasoning. For example, it is acknowledged that clinical/professional reasoning is affected by a number of factors, including the order in which information is obtained. Humans tend to favour the hypotheses they have developed and can tend to overemphasize information that supports a favoured hypothesis and disregard information that does not support or refutes it. By using a model of practice, therapists can be guided to overcome a tendency to collect information according to routines and habits that are not comprehensive (or have 'blind spots') and to be more systematic in the sources and type of information they collect. Models of practice can also help them to identify gaps in their knowledge and actively seek out information they might not have, rather than being overly influenced by the information they have already acquired.

Finally, models of practice provide guidance about what could *ideally* be done. As stated, they are comprehensive and holistic. However, they also aim to guide practice beyond one particular practice (and organizational) setting. Because it is not possible for them to be context specific, they can be very useful in guiding occupational therapists to work out more 'ideal' solutions. However, they cannot possibly take into account the specific context in which any individual therapist finds him- or herself. Therefore, it requires professional reasoning on the part of the occupational therapist to determine what can be done in that particular practice setting, given the constraints of factors such as time, resources, role expectations and the skills of the therapist.

## CONCLUSION

Professionals draw upon complex and extensive knowledge bases for their practice. As professionals are expected to be able to think and act in practice, these knowledge bases cover different types of knowledge that support different aspects of professional practice. Two of these types of knowledge are theory (episteme) and practical knowledge (phronesis). Professionals also have to use their knowledge of themselves and their skills and abilities.

A range of different terminology is used to categorize theory in occupational therapy. The use of these terms depends on the way that different levels of theory are categorized by the author. Some of the major ways that terminology is used to refer to theory and its relationship to practice were reviewed in this chapter. In this book, we focus on those levels of theory that aim primarily to guide practice. We refer to this level of theory as models of practice. Models of practice aim to guide occupational therapists to put into action the profession's unique understanding of occupation and its relationship to everyday life.

Being able to put occupational therapy into action not only requires knowledge of the profession's unique perspective, but also an understanding of the context within which that action must take place and the ability to identify and choose from a range of potential actions. In this chapter, we highlighted that occupational therapists work with particular people in specific contexts. We also emphasized that, while models of practice aim to guide practice, occupational therapists are required to use their professional reasoning skills to make decisions in practice. As Kielhofner (1995) stated, "Theory can never tell therapists, in advance, exactly what should be done in the context of therapy" (p. 1). Models of practice provide a framework within which to reason, but occupational therapists also require the ability to reason and make decisions about action.

In Chapter 2 we present a model of context-specific professional reasoning. Both occupational therapists and their clients exist within specific contexts. For occupational therapists, these contexts shape their roles and purposes and include the social, political and organizational contexts in which they work. They also exist as members of their professional communities of practice. Models of practice are artefacts of this community and help occupational therapists to determine their role as an occupational therapist within a particular organization and with particular clients. Because they are based in the philosophical perspectives of the profession, models of practice combine with professional reasoning to guide practitioners in determining how to be an occupational therapist in a particular context with particular clients and in combining thinking and action.

## REFERENCES

Aristotle, 1975. The Nicomachean ethics, Books I-X, (D. Ross, Trans.). Oxford University Press, London (Original work published 1925).

Carr, W., 1995. For education: Towards critical educational inquiry. The Open University, Buckingham, UK.

Cole, M.B., Tufano, R., 2008. Applied theories in occupational therapy: A practical approach. Slack, Thorofare, NJ.

Crepeau, E.B., Boyt Schell, B.A., Cohn, E., 2009. Theory and practice in occupational therapy. In: Crepeau, E.B., Cohn, E.S., Boyt Schell, B.A. (Eds.), Willard & Spackman's occupational therapy, eleventh ed. Lippincott Williams & Wilkins, Baltimore, MD, pp. 428–434.

Duncan, E.A.S., 2006. An introduction to conceptual models of practice and frames of reference. In: Duncan, E.A.S. (Ed.), Foundations for practice in occupational therapy, fourth ed. Churchill Livingstone, Edinburgh, pp. 59–66.

Encarta, 2009. Pragmatism. http://encarta.msn.com/encyclopedia (accessed 18.08.09).

Higgs, J., Titchen, A., Neville, V., 2001. Professional practice and knowledge. In: Higgs, J., Titchen, A. (Eds.), Practice knowledge and expertise in the health professions. Butterworth Heinemann, Oxford, pp. 3–9.

Kessels, J.P.A.M., Korthagen, F.A.J., 1996. The relationship between theory and practice: Back to the classics. Educ. Researcher 25 (3), 17–22.

Kielhofner, G., 1995. A model of human occupation: Theory and application, second ed. Williams & Wilkins, Baltimore, MA.

Kielhofner, G., 1997. Conceptual foundations of occupational therapy, second ed. F.A. Davis, Philadelphia, PA.

Kielhofner, G., 2009. Conceptual foundations of occupational therapy, fourth ed. F.A. Davis, Philadelphia, PA.

Mattingly, C., Fleming, M.H., 1994. Clinical reasoning: forms of inquiry in a therapeutic practice. F.A. Davis, Philadelphia, PA.

Melton, J., Forsyth, K., Freeth, D., 2009. Using theory in practice. In: Duncan, E.A.S. (Ed.), Skills for practice in occupational therapy. Churchill Livingstone, Edinburgh, pp. 9–23.

Mosey, A.C., 1992. Applied scientific inquiry in the health professions: An epistemological orientation. American Occupational Therapy Association, Rockville, MD.

Polanyi, M., 1958. Personal knowledge: Towards a post-critical philosophy. Routledge & Kegan Paul, London.

Reel, K., Feaver, S., 2006. Models – terminology and usefulness. In: Davis, S. (Ed.), Rehabilitation: the use of theories and models in practice. Churchill Livingstone, Edinburgh, pp. 49–62.

Rolfe, G., 1998. The theory–practice gap in nursing: from research-based practice to practitioner-based research. J. Adv. Nurs. 28 (3), 672–679.

Rothstein, J.M., 2004. The difference between knowing and applying. Phys. Ther. 84 (4), 310–311.

Ryle, G., 1949. The concept of mind. Penguin Books, Harmondsworth, UK.

Sackett, D.L., 2000. Evidence based medicine: How to practice and teach EBM. Churchill Livingstone, Edinburgh.

Turpin, M., Higgs, J., 2010. Clinical reasoning and EBP. In: Hoffman, T., Bennett, S., Bennett, J., Del Mar, C. (Eds.), Evidence-based practice across the health professions. Churchill Livingstone, Melbourne, VIC, pp. 300–317.

Williams, L., 2005. In search of profession: a sociology of allied health. In: Germov, J. (Ed.), Second opinion: an introduction to health sociology. Oxford University Press, Melbourne, VIC.

Theory and practice

# Professional reasoning in context

2

## CHAPTER CONTENTS

The previous chapter explored different types of knowledge that professionals need to combine in order to make reasoned action. These include: (a) generalized, propositional knowledge that is often generated through research (episteme); (b) practical wisdom or professional craft knowledge, which is context-specific knowledge and relates to professional 'know-how' (phronesis); and (c) personal knowledge, which refers to a professional's knowledge of him- or herself as a person. Sackett's (2000) definition of evidence-based medicine was used to highlight the need to combine these different types of knowledge, which can be sourced from research, professional expertise and an awareness of patient/client values specifically and human concerns more generally, when making professional decisions.

We propose that, when combining all of these different types of knowledge to make decisions in specific contexts about particular clients (and considering their particular situations), models of practice can provide useful frameworks for organizing this varied information. As discussed in Chapter 1, occupational therapy theory is embedded within models of practice. Therefore, using them to combine information should help occupational therapists to seek and interpret information relevant to the profession's domain of concern.

The process of making professional decisions is influenced by context. The particular information that is sought by occupational therapists as a basis for

© 2011 Elsevier Ltd.
DOI: 10.1016/B978-0-7234-3494-8.00002-4

professional decision-making is not only shaped by the profession's domain of concern but also by the organizational and sociopolitical and cultural contexts within which the occupational therapist works. In this chapter, we refer to the literature on professional reasoning to better understand how occupational therapists navigate the process of making professional decisions in context. We present professional practice as a complex endeavour that requires judgement and critical reasoning, has ethical and practical dimensions, requires the logical use of 'facts' and generalized theoretical principles and occurs within the context of various communities of practice (both professional and organizational).

First, we explore the nature of professional practice in terms of its roles and expectations within Western society and the implications of these for professional reasoning and judgement. Second, we look at the practice of occupational therapy and present a historical account outlining how professional reasoning of occupational therapists has been investigated. Third, we propose a model of professional reasoning in context. Finally, we discuss the role of occupational therapy practice models in supporting professional reasoning.

## THE NATURE OF PROFESSIONAL PRACTICE

Occupational therapy is an important profession to society. Therefore, we commence our investigation of occupational therapy practice by considering the nature of professional practice more generally, beginning with the question: what does it mean to be a professional? According to Coles (2002), "society asks certain of its members to be professionals – to undertake certain tasks and perform certain roles that others cannot or will not do" (p. 3). This definition associates professionalism with social roles. Blair (1998) defined social role as guiding "the behaviour expected of an individual because of the social status occupied. For example, the behaviour expected of a health professional is specific expertise and proven ability to alter the illness or problem experienced by an individual" (p. 45). The social status that Blair mentions refers to both rights and obligations that are afforded on the basis of professional status.

Professionals like occupational therapists have a particular place in the social hierarchy, in that they are expected to perform tasks that others are not expected to perform and they have certain rights and obligations that others don't have. These rights include higher levels of financial remuneration and greater autonomy, for which society expects a higher level of expertise (obligations). This expertise relates to both skills and knowledge, in that particular professions often claim particular skills as exclusive to that profession and each profession has to demonstrate a particular and extensive knowledge base that others in society would not normally be expected to possess.

Professions also are afforded a level of autonomy, in that professions are not expected to detail everything they do and the reasoning behind those actions. This is partly because their reasoning is expected to be based on their extensive and particular knowledge base. It follows, then, that only others who have that same knowledge base can fully understand what is required of and appropriate to that particular profession. Therefore, professions are expected to engage in self-regulation (Coles, 2002).

Fish and Coles (1998) summed up well the status of professions in our society in the following statement:

> *Professionals are expected to be trustworthy, and in their turn they expect to receive the public's trust in them. In return professionals were prepared to undertake a lengthy period of education, which for many was particularly protracted in order for them to gain higher professional qualifications. They were prepared to commit considerable amounts of time and effort to their work. They did not watch the clock, or do it for the money. They did more than was asked of them. They went further than their contracts of employment. All because they felt it was right to do so. They were professionals. They stood somewhat apart from the rest of society. They took on a professional role. And in recompense for their personal commitment, society gave them professional status, a greater than average income. For this society expected high ethical standards of course, and the maintenance of confidentiality. The tacit agreement was this: society would trust professionals if they could be trusted. (p. 4)*

One way that professions demonstrate their trustworthiness is through the development of codes of ethics. These are statements of the types of behaviours that can be expected of members of that particular profession. Often professionals have access to privileged and sensitive information and they need to be able to assure society that they will deal with this information properly. In the context of the helping professions, this sensitive information usually relates to those receiving services, that is, clients. For example, clients often have to disclose very personal information about themselves to professionals and might have to participate in activities (such as having a person they don't know very well toilet or shower them) which require a higher level of physical contact than they would have with many people they know very well. Therefore, the codes of ethics of the helping professions detail the nature of the relationships in which professionals will and will not engage, how the rights of those people receiving services will be upheld and protected, and how information relating to those people will be handled. Consequently, codes of ethics usually contain statements about respecting clients and their privacy, maintaining relationships that have appropriate boundaries and that acknowledge the power imbalance inherent in professional relationships, and providing competent and effective services.

The purpose of codes of ethics is associated with the autonomy afforded and self-regulation expected of professions. While codes of ethics are necessary for outlining the behaviours that society should be able to expect from professionals, they only provide the foundation for self-regulation. The reputation of a profession is dependent on the degree to which the behaviours outlined in these codes are adhered to by individual professionals and the support for professional standards that is provided by regulatory bodies.

Another distinguishing feature of professional practice is the expectation that professionals are able use judgement to determine the best course of action in any given situation. As professionals are asked to deal with complex situations and problems, professionals are expected to use their judgement to discern *when* to apply *which* procedures (and when to refrain from applying those procedures). Often, the ability to use a high level of judgement is the criterion used to distinguish between professionals and technicians, where technicians might have a high level of technical expertise but not the knowledge base required to make such judgements. For professional practice, it is not enough to have only the technical skills required to carry out a particular range of procedures, although these skills are necessary. Professionals are expected to use their extensive knowledge and apply this knowledge in different settings to address problems that present in a particular situation.

The primary purpose of this expert judgement is to make decisions about a course of action. Society expects professionals to be able to make decisions about action. Carr (1995) emphasized that professional action is not 'right' in an absolute sense (of there being a right thing to do) but that it is right when it is "*reasoned* action that can be defended discursively in argument and justified as morally appropriate to the particular circumstances in which it was taken" (p. 71, italics in original). Higgs et al. (2001) referred to professional practice as requiring "thoughtful action" (p. 5) in which professionals need to be able to take action to relieve or improve problems that clients encounter. Thus, the purpose of using professional judgement is to determine action that is reasoned and thoughtful.

Professionals are expected to use their profession's knowledge base as a foundation for their judgements. Having a unique knowledge base is central to the notion of profession. As Higgs et al. (2001) described:

> A 'profession' is an occupational group that is able to claim a body of knowledge distinctive to itself, whose members are able to practice competently, autonomously and with accountability, and whose members contribute to the development of the profession's knowledge base. In the emergence of the health occupations as professions, propositional knowledge, derived from research and scholarship, was sought to provide the foundation of the professions' knowledge base and their theory for practice, and to establish the professions' status and credibility. (p. 4)

Traditionally, the ability to make professional judgements about appropriate action has been conceptualized as a process of applying theory, given that professionals are expected to possess extensive theoretical knowledge. However, this assumption has been questioned. Mattingly and Fleming (1994) stated of occupational therapists:

> While [they] sometimes speak of clinical reasoning as the application of theory to practice, this is a deceptive statement. A grounding in theory is essential for expert practice but does not guarantee such practice. One cannot do without such grounding, but it, alone, will not yield good clinical interventions, because theoretical reasoning differs from practical reasoning. (p. 9)

If, as Mattingly and Fleming (1994) argued, theory is essential for professional practice but insufficient to guarantee expert practice, then professionals might need a range of different types of knowledge and skills to support their practice. As professionals need to both make judgements and engage in reasoned action, they need information that supports them to gain an expert understanding of the overall situation as well as information that provides the basis for judgements about action.

In Chapter 1, we discussed three different types of knowledge that professionals use, which could be categorized as either propositional or non-propositional knowledge. All three types of knowledge are necessary for expert and well-reasoned professional practice. By understanding the general principles conveyed through propositional knowledge, professionals can generate an understanding of the specific situation from a broader perspective of how things are structured and operate (e.g. using knowledge bases such as anatomy, physiology, psychology, sociology), knowledge of the general effectiveness of particular interventions (using 'evidence' generated from systematic research such as randomized controlled trials) and the perspective generated by theories that underpin the particular profession to which the professional belongs. However, they also need non-propositional knowledge. Context-specific professional craft knowledge underpins their ability to judge what action is required in the specific situation and to know how to carry out that action. Personal knowledge is used for the interpersonal aspects of professional action, as the ability to listen to, communicate with and develop a professional relationship with clients is well recognized as an essential component of professional practice (Price, 2009).

In summary, to be a professional means to fulfil a social role. This comes with social expectations as well as social privileges. The expectations include ethically sound behaviour and the ability to make well-reasoned and thoughtful judgements about action. These expert judgements are expected to be based on a unique and extensive base of propositional knowledge. Increasingly, it is recognized that well-reasoned judgements also rely on non-propositional knowledge such as professional craft knowledge and personal knowledge.

## COMMUNITIES OF PRACTICE

While professional practice is situated within the context of a society that expects its professionals to be able to provide services that are not expected of others, it also exists within the historical and social context of a particular profession. Carr (1995) made the point that to practise as a professional:

> is always to act within a tradition, and it is only by submitting to its authority that practitioners can begin to acquire the practical knowledge and standards of excellence by means of which their own practical competence can be judged. (pp. 68–69)

Professionals are expected to develop expertise in a particular type of practice, but how does this occur? A traditional approach to this question is to focus on the knowledge and skills that characterize the practice of a particular profession. From this perspective, teaching student and novice professionals the knowledge and skills of the profession is the logical approach to the development of expertise. The structure of many professional courses requires students to demonstrate their acquisition of the knowledge base that underpins practice as well as those skills deemed necessary for that particular kind of practice. In addition, practice educators recognize the importance of practical experience in developing expertise (Evenson, 2009). Consequently, bodies such as the World Federation of Occupational Therapists outline what they conceive as minimum standards for professional education that include a minimum number of hours of practice-based learning (Hocking & Ness, 2002). Professional expertise is based on practical experience as well as the acquisition of knowledge and skills.

Sociocultural approaches to learning provide a useful way of explaining the development of professional expertise. These approaches "explain learning and the development of expertise in terms of an individual's enculturation into the cultural practices or activities of their society and, more particularly, into the subcultures or communities of that society" (Walker, 2001, p. 24). Lave and Wenger (1991) used the term 'communities of practice' (p. 29) to refer to the communities to which individuals belong and within which they engage in situated or context-specific learning. Individual professionals develop expertise by participating in the cultural practices of the community of practice (in this case the profession, but they could also refer to multidisciplinary teams that the occupational therapist works in). Cultural practices include actions that are routine within a particular group. Often the practices are so accepted and routine that they might not be noticed by the group itself. As such, these practices are often described as tacit or embedded in practice, because they are probably not usually put into words or commented on.

From this perspective, professional learning is not simply the acquisition of skills but involves a transformation in the way that an individual participates in their community of practice. This process of transformation is a mutual one. As Walker (2001) explained, "As individuals are enculturated into the practices of their society and communities, they are transformed by the experience, and simultaneously may transform the community's practices" (p. 24). Participating in cultural practices contributes to a transformation in the professional's identity and action. The transformation of practices that results from such participation also contributes to the growth and development of the profession. In many ways, the models reviewed in this book could be seen as *cultural artefacts* (Iwama, 2007, p. 185) and reviewing how they have changed over time demonstrates one type of transformation that has occurred in the profession of occupational therapy. As Walker noted, cultural practices are interconnected but "have their own histories and trajectories and are part of, and linked to, other practices" (p. 24).

Professional relationships appear to be important for learning cultural practices. Parboosingh (2002) proposed that the interactions and relationships that professionals have with each other are important to the learning that occurs through participation in communities of practice. He stated, "the experiences of practitioners suggest that interacting with peers and mentors in the workplace provides the best environment for learning that enhances professional practice and professional judgment" (p. 230). In occupational therapy, Unsworth (2001) also proposed that "novice therapists could benefit from spending more time reflecting on the therapy process, and discussing their therapy with expert colleagues" (p. 163). Coles (2002, p. 7) explained that such learning also changes practice by leading to the "critical reconstruction of practice", that is, developing and enriching practice traditions, rather than just reproducing current practice.

In summary, practice expertise or practical wisdom is built through participation in communities of practice and enhances professional practice and professional judgement. Professional expertise requires extensive and relevant propositional knowledge bases and the ability to exercise professional judgements in order to make decisions about the best course of action in a particular situation. Practical wisdom is highly context-specific. Professionals have to combine and evaluate different types of knowledge in order to make practice decisions. A variety of terms are used to refer to the processes they use to do this. These terms include professional reasoning, clinical reasoning, professional or clinical judgement, and professional or clinical decision-making. Now we turn to an exploration of professional reasoning in occupational therapy.

## OCCUPATIONAL THERAPY PROFESSIONAL REASONING

Coles (2002) defined professional practice as "the exercise of discretion, on behalf of another, in a situation of uncertainty" (p. 4). This definition points to the requirement for professionals to make judgements that will affect their clients and that such judgements are often made in conditions of uncertainty. The uncertainty of the situations in which professional practice takes place (Coles, 2002; Hunink et al., 2001) and the need for professional judgements are well recognized (Higgs & Jones, 2008).

As professionals, occupational therapists need to be able to make well-reasoned decisions about their professional action. In this section of the chapter, we discuss professional reasoning from a historical perspective, explore the nature of occupational therapy practice as requiring art, science and action, and propose a model for conceptualizing context-specific reasoning in occupational therapy.

### HISTORICAL VIEW OF PROFESSIONAL REASONING IN OCCUPATIONAL THERAPY

In occupational therapy, research into the process of thinking and making judgements in practice has generally adopted the term clinical reasoning. This term was used in medicine and the early conceptualizations of occupational therapy reasoning were largely influenced by that research. The initial clinical reasoning research in occupational therapy was conducted by Joan Rogers and her colleagues in the early 1980s (Rogers, 1983; Rogers & Masagatani, 1982). At that time, clinical reasoning was generally understood from the perspective of artificial intelligence, with its focus on acquiring and managing information. Therefore, clinical reasoning was described as a process involving the acquisition and interpretation of cues (information) and the generation and testing of hypotheses (about what the cues might mean and their implications for professional action). This way of thinking often was called logico-deductive reasoning, because the emphasis was on a logical process of systematically collecting, combining and interpreting information in the light of established theories (i.e. deducing meaning).

Research funded by the AOTA and conducted by Cheryl Mattingly and Maureen Hayes Fleming in the late 1980s has dominated subsequent thinking about clinical reasoning in occupational therapy. Mattingly and Fleming (1994) presented their observations of clinical practice in a large rehabilitation facility in the United States of America. They argued that reasoning could be categorized into four different types: procedural, interactive, conditional and narrative. This work was influential, not only through the results of their methodologically rigorous research, but through introduction of the idea that occupational therapists might have multiple ways of reasoning. Prior to their work, clinical reasoning in occupational therapy had been conceptualized (in the same way as medicine) only as a hypothetico-deductive process. In contrast, Mattingly and Fleming stated that, in occupational therapy, "different modes of thinking are employed for different purposes and in response to particular features of the clinical problem complex" (p. 17).

Using the term *the three track mind*, Mattingly and Fleming (1994; also see Fleming, 1991) observed that occupational therapists switched between the first three of the four types so rapidly that they appeared to be using them simultaneously. First they used procedural reasoning, which relates to situations in which therapists focused on defining problems and considering intervention possibilities. They thought about the *procedures* they might use to remediate the person's problems with functional performance. Second, an interactive mode of reasoning was used when the therapist wanted to "interact with and better understand the person" (p. 17). This understanding appeared to be particularly important when the therapist wanted to tailor their intervention for the particular client. The third type of reasoning that formed part of the three track mind was conditional reasoning, which is "a complex form of social reasoning, [that] is used to help the patient in the difficult process of reconstructing a life that is now permanently changed by injury or disease" (p. 17). It is interesting to read their comments about this type of reasoning because it alludes to the problems of trying to put language to practice when much of it is embedded within practice and not generally put into words. They wrote, "The concept of conditional reasoning is perhaps the most elusive notion in our proposed theory of multiple modes of thinking. Yet we are firmly, if intuitively, convinced that there is a third form of reasoning that many experienced therapists used. This reasoning style moves beyond specific concerns about the person and the physical problems and places them in broader social and temporal contexts." (p. 18.) In addition to the three modes of reasoning that contributed to the three track mind, the final form of reasoning these authors proposed was a narrative mode of reasoning in which occupational therapists swapped stories and engaged others in discussing puzzling situations. They suggested that this storytelling also served as a way to enlarge each other's "fund of practical knowledge" vicariously (p. 18).

In 1993, Schell and Cervero published an "integrative review" of the clinical reasoning literature at the time. As a number of terms had been used to discuss different aspects of clinical reasoning that could be categorized as predominantly hypothetico-deductive, such as diagnostic reasoning (Rogers, 1983) and procedural reasoning (Mattingly, 1991; Mattingly & Fleming, 1994), Schell and Cervero grouped these together and labelled the category "scientific reasoning". This term was adopted by other authors and used frequently in subsequent publications relating to clinical reasoning in occupational therapy. Possibly taking Mattingly's and Fleming's lead of proposing that occupational therapists use multiple modes of reasoning, Schell and Cervero proposed an additional category of reasoning, which they called "pragmatic reasoning". Pragmatic reasoning referred to those times when occupational therapists thought about what actually *could* be done, given the practice resources available in the situation, the broader organizational and political context and the wishes of the client. They also made reference to ethical reasoning, where occupational therapists attended to what *should* be done (Rogers, 1983).

These earlier studies were followed by a continued interest in clinical reasoning over the following years, with a number of journals publishing special editions on clinical reasoning in the mid 1990s. More recently, Unsworth (2005) undertook research to test the presence of the various types of reasoning that had been described. She concluded that occupational therapists do appear to use procedural, interactive, conditional and pragmatic reasoning (proposing that this last one was more related to the influence of the practice environment than to the therapist's personal philosophy – both of which had been proposed by Schell & Cervero earlier) and that occupational therapists also seemed to use a process of linking the current situation to broader principles. She called this process "generalization reasoning" and proposed that it was a subcategory of each of the other types of reasoning. Examples of generalization reasoning included making generalizations about people with a particular medical diagnosis and general principles relating to the provision of services (both in that organization or service context and relating more specifically to occupational therapy interventions).

## ART, SCIENCE AND ACTION

When discussing the complexity of practice, Mattingly and Fleming (1994) observed that occupational therapy was a profession between two cultures, the culture of biomedicine and its own professional culture. As they stated, "one of the most interesting features of occupational therapy practice is that it tends to deal with functional problems that fall nicely within biomedicine (treating physical injuries with specific treatment techniques), as well as problems going far beyond the physical body, encompassing social, cultural, and psychological issues that concern the meaning of illness or injury to a person's life" (p. 37). In labelling this observation, they referred to occupational therapy as a "two-body practice" (p. 37) where occupational therapists attend to both physical and phenomenological bodies.

As discussed in the Introduction, a biomedical perspective most highly values the scientific method as a way of generating knowledge. It is characterized by a focus on the physical body and dominated by the body-as-machine metaphor. Mattingly and Fleming (1994) contrasted this with a phenomenological perspective, which focuses on the experience of illness rather than the physical impairment. This experiential dimension is often referred to as the lived body (referring to the body as it is lived or experienced) and is consistent with the concept of subjective experience, which is part of a biopsychosocial approach.

While different professions attend to both perspectives to various degrees, Mattingly and Fleming (1994) commented that occupational therapists are seemingly unique among the health professions by attending to both features equally. Similarly, Blair and Robertson (2005) claimed that occupational therapy lies on "what might be considered to be a 'professional fault line' between health and social care" (p. 272), whereby they seemed to be equating healthcare with a scientific, biomedical approach and social care with a perspective more concerned with people's social and personal welfare. This dual orientation might contribute to the complexity of reasoning required in occupational therapy.

In occupational therapy, the process required for such dual attention has long been referred to as art and science. A familiar definition of occupational therapy refers to the "art and science of man's [sic] participation…" (AOTA, 1972, p. 204). The equal importance of both perspectives was emphasized by Turpin (2007), who stated, "When occupational therapists refer to the paired concepts of art and science, they express their moral dissatisfaction with being constrained by either. In isolation, art somehow seems too soft and unquantifiable and science too hard and unyielding. The pairing of art and science expresses the complexity of occupational therapy; we are not one thing, but many" (p. 482). Kielhofner (1997) explained the implications of this dual perspective for clinical reasoning by saying, "Managing the intersection of scientific understanding and judgement with artful practice is challenging work. It requires occupational therapists to balance different ways of knowing and thinking in action" (p. 88).

Also contributing to an understanding of its complexity is the observation that action, observation and interpretation are integral to occupational therapy reasoning. Mattingly and Fleming (1994) observed that occupational therapists don't just reason and then act but reason *through* action and observation. They ask their clients to do certain things in order to observe them (to collect or interpret information) and they engage in action themselves in order to collect information to help them understand how people are performing their everyday occupations. This understanding then informs further action to collect more specific information or to test their judgements about interventions or their understanding of the situation.

Reasoning in action is not simply a process of trial and error, but a specific and targeted process. Mattingly and Fleming (1994) concluded that occupational therapists compare their observations with their pre-existing "stock of basic knowledge" (p. 322) in order to make interpretations and inferences. As they stated, "observations become information only if they can be used against a backdrop of prior knowledge" (p. 322). It may be that the process Unsworth (2005) called "generalization reasoning" is the same as the linking of observations made in specific situations to a stock of prior knowledge. All three types of knowledge outlined by Higgs et al. (2001) – propositional, professional craft and personal knowledge – can contribute to this stock of prior knowledge. As occupational therapists gain experience, learning from these experiences is added to this stock of knowledge. This explains why expert occupational therapists form their judgements on the basis of "smaller bits of information" (Mattingly & Fleming, p. 323) and less (but more targeted) action than novice occupational therapists. They have a more extensive (and probably more organized) stock of knowledge from which to draw when planning action.

## A MODEL FOR PROFESSIONAL REASONING IN CONTEXT

While models of practice provide a broad framework to assist occupational therapists in conceptualizing their work, professional reasoning is needed to determine what to do in a particular practice situation with a particular client.

In order to support the *use* of models in practice, in this section, we present the Model of Context-specific Professional Reasoning (MCPR), a model for conceptualizing occupational therapy reasoning in context. While there are other models of professional reasoning (e.g. see Schell, 2009), we propose that other models pay insufficient explicit attention to context. For example, in describing her ecological model of professional reasoning (Schell, 2009), the only statement pertaining to context was Schell's statement, "the therapist and the client function within a community of practice that shapes the nature, scope, and trajectory of the therapy process" (p. 324). In this chapter, we have discussed how a community of practice influences practice. However, the encounter between both clients (whether individuals or collectives) and therapists occurs within a broader organizational, legislative and policy, and cultural context. The Model of Context-specific Professional Reasoning conceptualizes professional reasoning as highly contextualized.

As discussed in the chapter so far, occupational therapists, as professionals, fulfil socially recognized roles. Within these roles, they have to make complex professional judgements under conditions of uncertainty. In occupational therapy, the complexity of decision-making relates to both the complex reasoning required of professionals in general and to the equal attention that occupational therapists pay to both physical and lived bodies.

Occupational therapy professional practice also requires both thinking and action. Occupational therapy practice includes a process of reasoned action, in which practitioners act and ask others to act in order to observe and collect information. They interpret this information using their stock of prior knowledge, which includes both context-specific information and general-ized knowledge. This information is collected in a range of different ways (e.g. formal and informal assessments, interviews and discussions with clients, accessing medical information and reports from other professionals) and, as Mattingly and Fleming (1994) noted, occupational therapists seem to observe constantly. Diverse information needs to be integrated and synthesized to enable practitioners to make judgements about the services they might offer. This synthesis is not necessarily easy as the information practitioners collect can be conflicting and difficult to interpret and combine.

Occupational therapy reasoning shares features with the reasoning of other health professionals. Turpin and Higgs (2010) stated that professional reasoning: (1) is inherently complex in nature; (2) is embedded within decision–action cycles; (3) is influenced by contextual factors; (4) requires collaborative decision-making; and (5) evolves into multiple ways of reason-ing as expertise increases.

Higgs and Jones (2008) also identified three core dimensions of clinical reasoning and three interactive/contextual dimensions. The core dimensions are: (1) discipline-specific knowledge, both propositional and non-propositional; (2) cognition, whereby practitioners compare more objective clinical information with their existing stock of discipline-specific and personal knowledge and interpret it with regard to client needs and preferences; and (3) metacognition. In discussing metacognition, they stated, "[practitioners] identify limitations in the quality of information obtained, inconsistencies or unexpected findings; it [metacognition] enables them to monitor their reasoning and practice, seek-ing errors and credibility; it prompts them to recognize when their knowledge or skills are insufficient and remedial action is needed" (p. 5). In recognition of the increasing emphasis on client-centred practice and consumer engagement in health, they included the additional dimensions of mutual decision-making, the decision-maker's interaction with the context and the impact of the task or problem on the reasoning.

While professionals acquire discipline-specific knowledge, it is well recognized that they also develop a stock of context-specific knowledge the longer they work in one place or area of practice. This was outlined in work on the development of expertise (Benner, 1984; Dreyfus & Dreyfus, 1986), which proposes that professionals develop expertise through experience in particular contexts. Consequently, when they practice in a different area, people with expertise in a previous area use the thinking strategies associated with the less experienced stages until they develop experience in the new area. This suggests that context-specific knowledge is fundamental to expertise.

To summarize, the work on professional reasoning generally (and that of occupational therapists more specifically) suggests that professionals:

1. Acquire a stock of different types of knowledge including propositional and non-propositional discipline-specific knowledge and context-specific knowledge. They continually add to all of these types of knowledge as they gain practical experience and theoretical knowledge.
2. Collect information pertaining to the client and his/her/their unique situation. This can be done through a range of processes such as formal and informal assessments, observing clients performing everyday occupations (could be an individual or group of people such as workers doing what they normally do), reviewing written documents pertaining to the client (e.g. medical records, reports), discussing the situation with other professionals (e.g. other professionals who are or have been working with the client), and cycles of action and observing and interpreting the results of that action.
3. Use cognitive processes to compare information that they collect about the client and the client's situation with their stock of knowledge (propositional and non-propositional discipline- and context-specific knowledge), make interpretations, determine what other information they might need, and plan and evaluate further action (and cycles of action).
4. Use metacognitive processes to evaluate the quality and utility of the information available and to reflect upon and evaluate their own reasoning processes (and monitor and correct errors) and skills.

Figure 2.1 is a diagrammatic representation of our Model of Context-specific Professional Reasoning (MCPR). In this model, we have purposely centred the reasoning on the interaction between a professional and another person, to emphasize that professional reasoning is ultimately context- and person-specific. That is, it occurs in a particular time and place, with particular people and in the context of particular relationships. It may include direct contact with a person or reference to the image of a type of person (e.g. when preparing resources for populations and subpopulations).

The choice of the word *person/s* might appear to invite the criticism that the model only applies to work with individual clients, but this is not the case. The term person was selected, rather than 'client', because the model distinguished

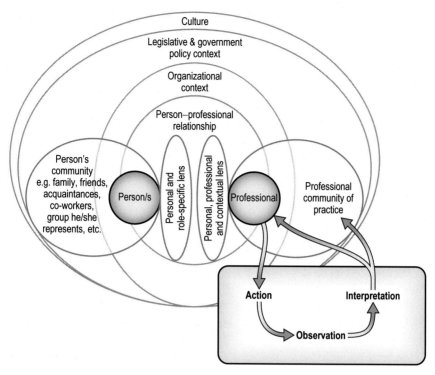

FIG 2.1   Model of Context-specific Professional Reasoning (MCPR).

between the *focus* of the work (which often relates to clients) and the *interaction* with particular people (or images). Regarding the focus of the work, clients can include large and small groups or collectives of individuals as well as individuals and formal entities. For example, professionals such as occupational therapists might work with individual clients and their families, groups of individuals or entities such as organizations (e.g. government and non-government agencies) and companies (e.g. seeking to increase the safety of their employees). In some cases, the groups to which occupational therapists target work are whole populations or subpopulations (in such cases, these collectives are not generally referred to as clients). For example, an occupational therapist might be advocating for or engaged in developing policy that will provide needed resources to facilitate the participation of individuals with a disability (where they are working with images of people rather than specific clients).

Regardless of where the work is focused, it requires the professional to interact with *particular people*. These people might be clients themselves, people who have concerns for or connections with individual clients, or people who represent or are responsible for others in formal organizations such as an agency or corporation. The ultimate purpose of this interaction is for the professional to engage in action directly or to facilitate the action of others.

Regardless of whether occupational therapists are working directly with individuals, groups of individuals or through larger entities and collectives, they aim to make a positive impact upon the health and well-being of particular people – whether those people can be identified individually or are just

Professional reasoning in context

seen as part of a larger group, entity or population. For example, an occupational therapist might be working on rehabilitation with Mary Smith to reduce impairments or promote adaptation of aspects of her environment to improve wanted participation in life roles. Alternately, the occupational therapist might be working on a population-based health promotion campaign with the aim of improving the lives of people *like* Mary Smith (i.e. they can't identify which specific persons will benefit from the project).With these examples in mind, we conceptualize professional reasoning as aiming to impact upon particular people. We have used the term 'person' in the model to denote this.

Embedded within the model is the assumption that individuals exist within the context of relationships with others (both formal and informal). In that respect, the Model of Context-specific Professional Reasoning can be seen as influenced by a sociocultural approach. People live within broader social and cultural contexts. They are influenced by the people with whom they have direct relationships, larger communities of people and the ideas that are debated or taken-for-granted by those communities (often referred to as culture in its broader sense), and various ways that the society in which they live is structured and organized.

The model provides a diagrammatic representation of some of the contexts that surround the professional and the person/s with whom they are interacting to develop or provide a service. To simplify discussion of this complex situation, the diagram is divided into *foreground* and *background*. In the foreground of the diagram, are professionals and persons who bring particular perspectives to the encounter. Borrowing from Schell (2009), these are represented in the diagram as "lenses". Surrounding each person engaged in the encounter is a particular community that also influences his or her perspective. For all people, these include other people that influence their lives and perspectives. In addition, surrounding professionals are professional "communities of practice" (Lave & Wenger, 1991).

In the background of this encounter, there are various layers of social context that influence the encounter. In the diagram, these are represented as: (a) the person–professional relationship, which denotes the concept that relationships between people are more than the sum of the interactions of which they are constituted; (b) the organizational context, which aims to denote the particular practice environments in which the encounter occurs; (c) the context of legislation and policy that surrounds the encounter and within which all of the key characters in the encounter live; and (d) the culture of the society.

Figure 2.1 also includes a blue box with arrows. This component of the model makes explicit the reasoning in action that occupational therapists have been observed to use. Each aspect of the diagram is discussed in more detail.

## FOREGROUND FEATURES

In most practice scenarios, occupational therapists and persons/clients engage in some sort of relationship organized around the provision of a specific service. Both professionals and the person/s with whom they work bring their own particular perspectives to the encounter. We have borrowed the concepts of the personal and professional lenses from Schell (2009, p. 324) and added our own concept of the various roles the person and professional might be fulfilling and the professional's understanding of the specific context in which the encounter is taking place. Therefore, we have called these perspectives 'personal and role-specific' and 'personal, professional and contextual' lenses. The former role-specific lens might refer to lenses such as client, carer or policy developer. The latter denotes that professionals' perspectives are influenced by: (a) personal experiences and ways of understanding the world; (b) their identity and experience as a member of a particular profession (e.g. an occupational therapist) and the way they have internalized the values and beliefs of their professional community; and (c) their understanding and experience of their particular role within a specific practice context and the culture of that practice context.

These perspectives will be influenced by the personal qualities of each person. This 'personal lens' includes each person's beliefs, values, intelligence, embodied sense and abilities, and life experiences and living situation (Schell, 2009, p. 324). In addition, people bring perspectives that are shaped by their roles within the encounter. In many occupational therapy scenarios, the people engaging in the encounter in the role of client will bring particular expectations related to that role. For example, they might have particular expectations for the professional's level of expertise and the degree of collaboration that should occur. The occupational therapist will also bring expectations relating to his or her own behaviour and that of clients within the particular practice context in which the encounter is taking place. In addition, a professional's role will be shaped by the particular practice context in which the encounter occurs. How they approach and perceive the specific situation will be influenced by their knowledge of what is done in that organization and how.

Both the person and the professional are also influenced by their respective communities. In the case of people receiving services (clients), they will have a range of experiences and formal and informal relationships with the people connected to them. These will all influence the perspectives they bring to the encounter – both their personal perspective and their expectations relating to the role of client – and the degree to which they are likely to follow recommendations that the professional might make. These relationships will also influence the personal and material resources that are available to clients and will impact upon what *can* be done (pragmatic reasoning regarding intervention/service delivery options). For example, the number of people a family's financial resources needs to support will impact upon whether services that carry a financial cost can be offered and how often the relevant family members can afford to attend the service (i.e. cost of service, transport, time off from work, etc.). An intervention for a disabled person living in a group home might need commitment from support workers to carry out or supervise what has been recommended. Any recommendations for change to workplaces will need to be appropriate to the culture of the workplace (management and workers) and the processes required to undertake their core business.

As with their clients, professionals are also surrounded by their own communities, which will influence their personal perspectives. In addition to this, they are part of communities of practice, such as the local, national and international community of occupational therapists, which influence their professional perspective. As a profession, occupational therapy has its own unique knowledge base, values and perspectives and these influence the perspectives each professional will bring to an encounter with clients. It influences what kinds of information they seek and how they collect it, how they interpret information, and what kinds of interventions and services they feel they can offer.

## BACKGROUND FEATURES

So far we have discussed the part of the diagram that is foregrounded. Now we turn to the *background* of a broader, multilayered context within which an encounter occurs. In the model, we have identified four of the major layers of context that surround any encounter between professionals and service users.

The first is the *relationship* between the people involved in the encounter. While each individual will bring their particular lens to the encounter, the relationships that develop between the various people involved will also influence the process and outcome of the encounter. Relationship is specified as a particular background feature because the relationships that people develop can influence the decisions that are able to be made. For example, an occupational therapist might be working with a particular organizational client. He or she might have built a facilitatory relationship with a particular manager and be able to make certain recommendations and have a high level of confidence that they would be implemented. However, if a new person came into that position, because they would have a different relationship, the recommendations the occupational therapist might make are likely to differ.

The importance of relationships between professionals and clients is well recognized as affecting the outcome of their encounters (Price, 2009). Examples of these person–professional relationships include relationships with individual clients and their significant others, with groups of clients, with people in management or supervisory positions who are responsible for a group of workers or the management practices of a company, and with elders or leaders of particular community groups. These relationships are central to occupational therapy philosophy as occupational therapists aim to work *with* people rather than doing things to them. It is through these different types of relationships that they aim to influence the health and well-being of individuals, groups and populations.

The next layer of context relates to the *organization* in which the person–professional interaction occurs. We have called it organizational context because most occupational therapy work is undertaken within a particular practice context. Whether the occupational therapist is being paid or doing the work in a voluntary capacity, they are usually either providing services directly through particular organizations or working with particular organizations to influence their provision of services and resources. The term organization is defined as "a body of persons organized for some end or work" (Macquarie Dictionary, 1985, p. 1202). We are using the term in this broad way to denote a range of different types of organizations such as government and non-government agencies, corporations, service delivery organizations, incorporated bodies, etc.

Organizations are important to consider as a context in which the person–professional encounter occurs (and therefore where professional reasoning is required) because they have a particular culture that influences *what* work is done and *how* it is done. This culture shapes occupational therapy practice at subconscious and conscious levels. That is, occupational therapists might develop routine ways of seeing and doing things in a particular context or they might be consciously aware of the constraints and demands that the practice environment places on their practice. Organizations are established for a particular purpose and there is an expectation that the people working for them or with them will be instrumental in fulfilling that purpose. These expectations will help shape the professional lens. Similarly, clients and others will come with particular expectations about that organization regarding the type and quality of services or assistance provided. These expectations form part of their role–specific lens.

The next layer of context relates to the society in which the encounter takes place. Larger societies have formal *legislative and government processes* that determine the rules of that society. In parliamentary democracies, laws are made through acts of Parliament and enforced by legal processes (e.g. courts) and regulators, and organizations such as police forces. Subgroups might also exist in societies, in which persons hold recognized positions and provide leadership and governance to that subgroup such as elders of indigenous groups. Both professionals and the people they work with have to abide by the laws of the society and will be influenced by the policies (and subsequent services and practices) developed and/or funded by the government.

The final layer, which influences all of those layers within it, is the *culture* of the society. Cultural (and subcultural) beliefs and practices pervade the lives of people and influence their behaviour. They also influence the expectations and social mores relating to relationships between professionals and clients, as well as the organizations that are developed (and allowed) and the laws and policies that are created. Cultural beliefs and practices are often held and enacted at a subconscious level, as people who have grown up in those cultural contexts will have internalized many values and beliefs. They become taken-for-granted assumptions. Often, people only become aware of those values and beliefs when they are confronted with situations that do not align with those values and beliefs. This might occur because of a particular event or circumstance, through moving from one culture to another, or when subcultural values do not align with those of the dominant culture or other subcultures.

## OCCUPATIONAL THERAPY REASONING AND ACTION

In addition to the multiple layers that surround person and professional, specific features of occupational therapy reasoning are included. This is presented in an additional box in the lower right of the diagram in Figure 2.1. This box is informed by Mattingly and Fleming's (1994) observations and interpretations of occupational therapy clinical reasoning. They emphasized that action is an integral part of occupational therapists' clinical reasoning and linked this to the profession's roots in the philosophical perspective of pragmatism (see the work of John Dewey, William James and Charles Sanders-Pierce). Other authors have also noted the influence of this tradition (Ikiugu, 2007).

Mattingly and Fleming (1994) noted that occupational therapists often reason through action – both their own and the action of others. Their study participants (occupational therapists) asked their clients to do something so that they could observe, with precision, how the client undertook these tasks. They also acted themselves (e.g. performed a formal assessment), in order to observe the outcome and, on the basis of their interpretations of those observations, make judgements. Consistent with the work of Higgs and colleagues, Mattingly and Fleming found that occupational therapists interpreted their observations by comparing them with their stock of knowledge (both theoretical and practice-based). This process of interpretation enabled them to make judgements about the clinical situation and to plan further action. The experience gained from these cycles of action, observation and interpretation was added to the professional's stock of knowledge and became part of the information against which further action cycles were interpreted.

The knowledge gained from these action cycles can also be used to change practice for more than just the individual practitioner. Walker (2001) emphasized that communities of practice both influence and are influenced by their members. This influence might occur in a formal sense as occupational therapists publish their work for others to read but it can also influence practice at the local level. Referring to physicians, Parboosingh (2002) claimed that these professionals "naturally form COP [communities of practice]" when working in the same area and that members of this community "contribute to the collective pool of evidence-based knowledge, drawn from the peer-reviewed literature, as well as tacit knowledge and practical wisdom derived from practice experience" (p. 231). The same could be said of occupational therapists. They spend time (formally and informally) sharing their knowledge and experiences and engaging in joint problem solving. Mattingly and Fleming (1994) stated that these processes expanded their stock of knowledge vicariously.

## OCCUPATIONAL THERAPY PROFESSIONAL REASONING AND MODELS OF PRACTICE

The Model of Context-specific Professional Reasoning highlights the complexity of factors that influence professional reasoning. These factors can relate to the personal qualities and experiences of the professional and his or her expectations about their professional role, the perspective of the discipline to which the professional belongs, personal aspects of the client/s and the expectations of the professional's role that they bring to the encounter, the nature of the encounter between clients and professionals and the organizational, legislative and government policy, and cultural contexts in which the client–professional encounter occurs (which all shape professional role expectations). All of these factors interact to create a unique situation for every client–professional encounter.

An important aspect of the model is the professional community of practice (which can be discipline-specific or multidisciplinary, e.g. multi- or transdisciplinary teams). Professionals develop their understanding of their particular professional discipline through professional socialization and the acquisition of the specific knowledge base unique to each profession. Professionals maintain their professional identities through access to and identification with their community of practice. This could be done directly by having contact with other members of the community of practice (e.g. through workshops and special interest groups or just through contact with co-workers) or less directly by reading publications produced by members of the community of practice and identifying with that community (e.g. by working with members of other professions and defining oneself as an occupational therapist and, therefore, different from the other professions because of particular professional values and perspectives that one shares with occupational therapy).

While professionals also belong to other communities of practice, such as multidisciplinary teams working together to provide a service to a particular subpopulation or group, the values and perspectives of the professional group to which they belong often shape their understandings in a variety of ways, of which they might not be aware because it "represents the unquestioned norm" (Trede & Higgs, 2008, p. 32) of their professional group. Unless they are able to make these assumptions overt, these norms can be difficult to examine and critique. Without such examination, the value of such norms cannot be established (either positively or negatively).

One of the ways that a shared vision of the occupational therapy community of practice is available is through its conceptual models of practice. Each of the models of practice discussed in this book presents a particular way of organizing and describing occupational therapy theoretical assumptions and values (the shared vision) for the purpose of guiding practice. In this regard they all share the perspectives and values that characterize occupational therapy as a profession and distinguish it from other professions. Therefore, the core of occupational therapy is encapsulated within the commonalities of the models. However, each model also emphasizes different aspects of the shared vision to different degrees. This variation probably relates to a combination of the different practice environments for which some of the models were originally developed, sociocultural differences relating to the country in which or for which they were developed, the time in occupational therapy's history in which they were developed or revised, and the particular philosophical perspectives that the authors chose to present or emphasize.

Trede and Higgs (2008) stated that, "models can be thought of as mental maps that assist practitioners to understand their practice" (p. 32). This is the way that we are conceptualizing them in this book. By exploring the different models of practice in detail in the one text, we hope to provide readers with a resource that helps them to compare and contrast the different occupational therapy models and to select models that support the professional reasoning they need to do in specific contexts at specific historical times. We also hope that this condensed presentation of occupational therapy models of practice helps readers to distil the essence of occupational therapy philosophy.

The chapters that follow present nine occupational therapy conceptual models of practice. They were all developed to guide practice by providing a systematic way to organize many of the core concepts of occupational therapy. The advantage of using conceptual models to guide practice is that they provide a systematic and comprehensive way to conceptualize practice. Often they are used in conjunction with other frameworks, which mostly provide greater detail about interventions and techniques relevant to a particular practice area. As discussed in Chapter 1, these are often referred to as frames of reference and frequently contain information that is not specific to occupational therapy. Conceptual models of practice, however, are specific to occupational therapy and contain the profession's core concepts. For each model, the core concepts and an overview of its history are described, and a memory aid is provided to facilitate use of the model in practice. In addition, the major references for each model are also provided As this book aims to provide an overview of some of the major occupational therapy conceptual models of practice, readers are encouraged to develop a more in-depth understanding of the models that they feel are most relevant to their own practices.

## SUMMARY

In this chapter, we discussed the nature of professional practice. We presented professions as groups that are recognized within society and are provided both obligations and privileges. Professions are afforded autonomy and, often, higher levels or remuneration whilst being expected to have a unique knowledge base, a code of ethics and engage in self-regulation. The profession to which an individual belongs operates as a community of practice in which the individual is surrounded by a larger professional body that shapes and is shaped by their learning about the culture of the profession.

Professionals are expected to fulfil particular roles in society. They generally work under conditions of uncertainty and are required to engage in professional reasoning to make judgements about what action/s to take in a particular circumstance. Occupational therapists value both art and science in their understanding of the needs of clients and their expectations about the interventions or services that they can offer. They place equal value on both when making decisions about what to do in their professional role.

Action is central to occupational therapy practice and an integral part of occupational therapists' decision-making. That is, they often think in and through action. Such action always occurs within a particular context, which shapes and is shaped by these decisions and actions. Thus, occupational therapy reasoning and decision-making is always context based.

In this chapter, we presented a model for understanding the context-specific nature of occupational therapy professional reasoning. The Model of Context-specific Professional Reasoning aims to assist occupational therapists to consider the range of contextual features that impact upon their reasoning. This model conceptualizes occupational therapy professional reasoning as:

(a) involving some form of interaction with a person (whether that be an individual, group or representative of an organizational client or a stakeholder or concerned person such as a family member);
(b) being shaped by the various lenses that each party brings to the encounter and the specific contexts surrounding each person;
(c) occurring within the context of a person–professional relationship, an organizational context, a legislative and government policy context and a culture; and
(d) including a cycle of action, observation and interpretation.

One of the ways that the occupational therapy community of practice shapes practice is through models of practice. These models are a level of theory that specifically aims to guide practice. In the chapters that follow, we present nine occupational therapy models of practice. For each, we present the major concepts as outlined in their most recent form, a discussion of their historical development, a list of major publications (these are not meant to be exhaustive but to provide a starting point for readers who wish to investigate the model in more detail), and a memory aid to assist occupational therapists when using the model in their practice.

## REFERENCES

AOTA, 1972. Occupational therapy: Its definition and function. Am. J. Occup. Ther. 26, 204.

Benner, P., 1984. From novice to expert: Excellence and power in clinical nursing practice. Addison-Wesley, Reading, MA.

Blair, S.E.E., 1998. Role. In: Jones, D., Blair, S.E.E., Hartery, T., Jones, R.K. (Eds.), Sociology and occupational therapy: An integrated approach. Churchill Livingstone, Edinburgh, pp. 41–53.

Blair, S.E.E., Robertson, L., 2005. Hard complexities – soft complexities: An exploration of philosophical positions related to evidence in occupational therapy. Br. J. Occup. Ther. 68 (6), 269–276.

Carr, W., 1995. For education: Towards critical educational inquiry. The Open University, Buckingham, UK.

Coles, C., 2002. Developing professional judgement. J. Contin. Educ. Health Prof. 22, 3–10.

Dreyfus, H., Dreyfus, S., 1986. Mind over machine: the power of human intuition and expertise in the era of the computer. The Free Press, New York.

Evenson, M., 2009. Fieldwork: The transition from student to professional. In: Crepeau, E.B., Cohn, E.S., Boyt Schell, B.A. (Eds.), Willard & Spackman's occupational therapy, eleventh ed. Lippincott Williams & Wilkins, Baltimore, MD, pp. 252–261.

Fish, D., Coles, C., 1998. Developing professional judgement in health care: Learning through the critical appreciation of practice. Butterworth Heinemann, Oxford.

Fleming, M.H., 1991. The therapist with the three-track mind. Am. J. Occup. Ther. 45, 1007–1014.

Higgs, J., Jones, M., 2008. Clinical decision making and multiple problem spaces. In: Higgs, J., Jones, M., Loftus, S., Christensen, N. (Eds.), Clinical reasoning in the health professions. Butterworth Heinemann, Philadephia, PA, pp. 3–17.

Higgs, J., Titchen, A., Neville, V., 2001. Professional practice and knowledge. In: Higgs, J., Titchen, A. (Eds.), Practice knowledge and expertise in the health professions. Butterworth Heinemann, Oxford, pp. 3–9.

Hocking, C., Ness, N.E., 2002. Minimum standards for the education of occupational therapists. World Federation of Occupational Therapists, Forrestfield, Australia.

Hunink, M.G.M., Glasziou, P.P., Siegel, J.E., Weeks, J.C., Pliskin, J.S., Elstein, A., et al., 2001. Decision making in health and medicine: Integrating evidence and values. Cambridge University Press, New York.

Ikiugu, M.N., 2007. Psychosocial conceptual practice models in occupational therapy: Building adaptive capability. Mosby, St Louis, MI.

Iwama, M., 2007. Culture and occupational therapy: meeting the challenge of relevance in a global world. Occup. Ther. Int. 4 (4), 183–187.

Kielhofner, G., 1997. Conceptual foundations of occupational therapy, second ed. F.A. Davis, Philadelphia, PA.

Lave, J., Wenger, E., 1991. Situated learning: legitimate peripheral participation. Cambridge University Press, New York.

Macquarie Dictionary, 1985. Revised ed. Macquarie Library, Dee Why, NSW.

Mattingly, C., 1991. The narrative nature of clinical reasoning. Am. J. Occup. Ther. 45 (11), 998–1005.

Mattingly, C., Fleming, M.H., 1994. Clinical reasoning: forms of inquiry in a therapeutic practice. F.A. Davis, Philadelphia, PA.

Parboosingh, J.T., 2002. Physician communities of practice: Where learning and practice are inseparable. J. Contin. Educ. Health Prof. 22, 230–236.

Price, P., 2009. The therapeutic relationship. In: Crepeau, E.B., Cohn, E.S., Boyt Schell, B.A. (Eds.), Willard & Spackman's occupational therapy, eleventh ed. Lippincott Williams & Wilkins, Baltimore, MD, pp. 328–341.

Rogers, J.C., 1983. Clinical reasoning: The ethics, science, and art. Am. J. Occup. Ther. 37, 601–616.

Rogers, J.C., Masagatani, G., 1982. Clinical reasoning of occupational therapists during the inital assessment of physically disabled patients. Occup. Ther. J. Res. 2, 195–219.

Sackett, D.L., 2000. Evidence based medicine: How to practice and teach EBM. Churchill Livingstone, Edinburgh.

Schell, B., 2009. Professional reasoning in practice. In: Crepeau, E.B., Cohn, E.S., Boyt Schell, B.A. (Eds.), Willard & Spackman's occupational therapy, eleventh ed. Lippincott Williams & Wilkins, Baltimore, MD, pp. 314–327.

Schell, B., Cervero, R., 1993. Clinical reasoning in occupational therapy: An integrative review. Am. J. Occup. Ther. 47, 605–610.

Trede, F., Higgs, J., 2008. Collaborative decision making. In: Higgs, J., Jones, M., Loftus, S., Christensen, N. (Eds.), Clinical reasoning in the health professions, third ed. Butterworth Heinemann, Oxford, pp. 31–41.

Turpin, M., 2007. The issue is… Recovery of our phenomenological knowledge in occupational therapy. Am. J. Occup. Ther. 61 (4), 481–485.

Turpin, M., Higgs, J., 2010. Clinical reasoning and EBP. In: Hoffman, T., Bennett, S., Bennett, J., Del Mar, C. (Eds.), Evidence-based practice across the health professions. Churchill Livingstone, Melbourne, VIC, pp. 300–317.

Unsworth, C., 2001. The clinical reasoning of novice and expert occupational therapists. Scand. J. Occup. Ther. 8, 163–173.

Unsworth, C., 2005. Using a head-mounted video camera to explore current conceptualizations of clinical reasoning in occupational therapy. Am. J. Occup. Ther. 59, 31–40.

Walker, R., 2001. Social and cultural perspectives on professional knowledge and expertise. In: Higgs, J., Titchen, A. (Eds.), Practice knowledge and expertise in the health professions. Butterworth Heinemann, Oxford, pp. 22–28.

# Occupational performance and adaptation models

3

## CHAPTER CONTENTS

© 2011 Elsevier Ltd.
DOI: 10.1016/B978-0-7234-3494-8.00003-6

This chapter includes a number of models that address occupational therapy from the perspective articulated most prominently in North America. While occupational therapy grew out of both British and North American movements, the way that occupational therapy has been conceptualized in North America has had a widespread influence on theory throughout the world. While a number of different occupational performance models had been developed in different Western countries (e.g. the Canadian Occupational Performance Model (OPM) (DNHW & CAOT, 1983)), two have been selected to demonstrate different aspects of this approach. These are occupational performance models from the USA and Australia. The first two models presented in this chapter are the Occupational Performance (OP) model (Pedretti & Early, 2001), and with it the Occupational Therapy Practice Framework (OTPF) (AOTA, 2008), and the Occupational Performance Model (Australia) (OPMA) (Chapparo & Ranka, 1997). These models are most frequently, although not exclusively, used in physical rehabilitation practice because these models include a detailed focus on the body and its component capacities. In addition, a third model, the Occupational Adaptation (OA) model (first published: Schkade & Schultz, 1992), is presented.

These three models are presented together in this chapter because they particularly use the language of 'science'. While this is evident in the two occupational performance models through their use of knowledge bases relating to the anatomy and physiology of the body, it is also evident in the extensive use of objective language (objectivity is highly valued in science) to label concepts in the Occupational Adaptation (OA) model. As discussed in the Introduction, over time the trend towards a more person-centred and less biomedical approach has characterized occupational therapy theory. Pedretti's OP model and Chapparo's and Ranka's OPMA provide a good example of this shift in emphasis, in that OP is more consistent with a biomedical approach through its focus on the physical body and performance components and OPMA with a biopsychosocial approach, which emphasizes subjective experience in addition to performance components.

The term *occupational performance* has been used widely in a range of occupational therapy publications, particularly in the late 1990s and early 2000s, and was often used interchangeably with other terms. As Christiansen and Baum (1997) explained, "The terms function or functional performance are often used in the medical literature to describe the ability of an individual to accomplish tasks of daily living. In an American Occupational Therapy Association (AOTA) position paper, Baum and Edwards (1995) observed that, when occupational therapists in the United States use the term function, they refer to an individual's performance of activities, tasks and roles during daily occupations (occupational performance)" (p. 5).

## OCCUPATIONAL PERFORMANCE MODEL

In this section, the Occupational Performance (OP) model, as articulated by Lorraine Williams Pedretti and her colleagues in the various editions of her well-known occupational therapy textbook, *Occupational Therapy: Practice Skills for Physical Dysfunction* (1981, 1985, 1990, 1996, 2001), is presented in detail in its most recent (2001) form. This model was chosen as a starting point for the chapter, because the concepts that are articulated in the model represent the way that occupational therapy was conceptualized in many Western countries over the course of the last century. Therefore, it is likely that many of the concepts in the model continue to influence occupational therapy theory and practice.

In this chapter, once the Occupational Performance model, as it was presented by Pedretti and Early (2001), has been outlined, more recent developments are discussed in a section on the historical description of the model's development. These include the Occupational Therapy Practice Framework (OTPF), first published in 2002 by the AOTA and now in its second edition (AOTA, 2008). While there are a range of occupational therapy models and frameworks published in the area of physical dysfunction, the OP model and the OTPF are both presented here because they flowed from or were associated with the official position of the AOTA (much of the Canadian work is discussed in Chapter 5). Pedretti's and Early's (2001) statement, "occupational performance terminology [used in the model] was defined and standardized in official documents of the AOTA" (p. 4) demonstrates that the OP model encapsulated the officially accepted view of the domain of concern of occupational therapy by the American Occupational Therapy Association at the time.

## MAIN CONCEPTS AND DEFINITIONS OF TERMS

Lorraine Williams Pedretti is the author most closely associated with articulating the OP model. She did not claim to have authored this model but explained that some components of the model "have always been the core of OT" (Pedretti & Early, 2001, p. 4) and other details were added by committees and task forces of the American Occupational Therapy Association during the 1970s. The diagram (1996, 2001) (see Figure 3.1) used to represent the model acknowledges that it is based on the uniform terminology for occupational therapists, which was published in three editions by the AOTA and was succeeded by the OTPF. Throughout the description of this model, the term

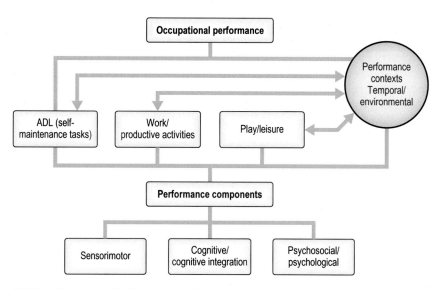

FIG 3.1   Occupational Performance model *(as presented by Pedretti & Early 1996, 2001).*

*patient* is used, as that is the term most often used in relation to this model. That is, the model used the term patient to refer to the subject of therapy, and for consistency, we do the same.

As the name suggests, the central aim in this model is to facilitate occupational performance. *Occupational performance* was defined as, "the ability to perform those tasks that make it possible to carry out occupational roles in a satisfying manner appropriate for the individual's developmental stage, culture, and environment" (Pedretti & Early, 2001, p. 5). Pedretti defined *occupational roles* as "the life roles that an individual holds in society" (1996, p. 3). Occupational roles develop in conjunction with the occupations in which people engage and include roles such as "pre-schooler, student, parent, homemaker, employee, volunteer, or retired worker" (2001, p. 5). Thus, the purpose of occupational performance is to be able to fulfil occupational roles.

The development of occupational performance is dependent upon sufficient opportunities to practice and learn the skills and abilities required to fulfil occupational roles and developmental tasks. The model provides a framework for aiding occupational therapists to systematically analyze the nature of the problems that are reducing the occupational performance of an individual. It comprises three elements: performance areas, performance components and performance contexts. The diagram provides the details of each of these elements and how they relate to occupational performance. Problems can arise that interfere with occupational performance. These problems might stem from "deficits in task learning experiences, performance components, or impoverished performance contexts" (Pedretti & Early, 2001, p. 5).

The *performance areas* are the first of the three elements described by the authors. The model outlines three performance areas into which activities are grouped. These are activities of daily living (ADL), work and productive activities, and play or leisure activities. Pedretti and Early (2001) explained, "ADL include the self-maintenance tasks of grooming, hygiene, dressing, feeding and eating, mobility, socialization, communication, and sexual expression. Work and productive activities include home management, care of others, educational activities, and vocational activities. Play and leisure include play exploration and play or leisure performance in age-appropriate activities." (p. 5.) It appears that, by explaining the performance areas first, their connection to occupational performance and occupational roles could be emphasized. In addition, Pedretti and Early stated, "intervention strategies must ultimately be directed to the patient's achievement in performance areas when a performance component (e.g. motor skill development) is being addressed" (p. 6). This emphasizes that, while the performance components provide details for occupational therapists that are particularly useful in planning rehabilitation interventions, occupational therapy intervention is for the purpose of enhancing the occupational performance required by an individual in each of the performance areas.

*Performance components* are "the learned developmental patterns of behaviour which are the substructure and foundation of the individual's occupational performance" (Pedretti & Early, 2001, p. 5). The components of performance are categorized in the following three groups: sensorimotor, cognitive and cognitive integration, and psychosocial and psychological components. According to this model, "adequate neurophysiological development and integrated functioning of the performance components are basic to an individual's ability to perform occupational tasks or activities in the performance areas" (pp. 5–6). The sensorimotor component includes three types of functions. These are sensory, neuromusculoskeletal and motor functions. The cognitive integration and cognitive components relate to the ability to use higher brain functions. The psychosocial and psychological components include those abilities required for social interaction and emotional processing. The model provides substantial detail about the nature of these performance components. These details have been listed in Table 3.1 for clarity.

The third element in the OP model is called *performance contexts*. The model acknowledges that occupational performance is conducted in a variety of contexts. Therefore, in order to gain a detailed understanding of an individual's occupational performance, occupational therapists need to know both how the abilities of the individual affect his or her performance and how the context in which occupations are performed influence that performance. Performance contexts are conceptualized as temporal and environmental. Pedretti and Early (2001) listed the following as examples of the temporal context: "the individual's age, developmental stage or phase of maturation, and stage in important life processes such as parenting, education, or career. . . [and] disability status (e.g., acute, chronic, terminal, improving, or declining) must also be considered" (p. 6). These examples suggest that, in this model, the temporal contexts appear to relate primarily to the individual.

Environmental dimensions of the performance contexts are considered under the categories of physical, social and cultural. As Pedretti and Early stated, "The physical environment includes homes, buildings, outdoors, furniture, tools, and other objects. Social environment includes significant others and social groups. Cultural environment includes customs, beliefs, standards of behaviour, political factors, and opportunities for education, employment, and economic support" (p. 6).

## INTERVENTION

Underlying the model are two key approaches to facilitating occupational performance: remediation and compensation. In a remediation approach, intervention is targeted towards improving performance components, with the assumption that such improvements will lead to enhanced occupational performance in the performance areas. A compensatory approach is used when remediation is not considered achievable or feasible. According to Pedretti and Early (2001), the latter approach "focuses on remaining abilities and aims to improve function by adapting or compensating for performance component deficits" (p. 6). They proposed that examples of this approach might include adapting the methods used to perform tasks, providing assistive devices or modifying the environment.

The model outlines four levels of intervention. As the main focus of this model is remediation, the four levels primarily categorize methods that could be used for the remediation of problems in performance components. The levels in sequence are adjunctive methods, enabling activities, purposeful activity and occupations. They represent an intervention continuum that "takes the patient through a logical progression from dependence to occupational

Table 3.1  *Performance components of the OP model*

| Sensorimotor components | | | Cognitive integration & cognitive components | Psychosocial and psychological components |
|---|---|---|---|---|
| **Sensory functions** | **Neuromusculoskeletal functions** | **Motor functions** | | |
| • Sensory awareness & processing & perceptual processing | • Reflex responses<br>• Range of motion<br>• Muscle tone<br>• Strength<br>• Endurance<br>• Postural control<br>• Postural alignment<br>• Soft-tissue integrity | • Gross coordination<br>• Crossing the midline<br>• Laterality<br>• Bilateral integration<br>• Motor control<br>• Praxis<br>• Fine coordination & dexterity<br>• Oral motor control | • Level of arousal<br>• Orientation<br>• Recognition<br>• Attention span<br>• Initiation of activity<br>• Termination of activity<br>• Memory<br>• Sequencing<br>• Categorization<br>• Concept formation<br>• Spatial operations<br>• Problem solving<br>• Learning<br>• Generalization | • Values<br>• Interests<br>• Self-concept<br>• Role performance<br>• Social conduct<br>• Interpersonal skills<br>• Self-expression<br>• Coping skills<br>• Time management<br>• Self-control |

performance to resumption of valued social and occupational roles" (Pedretti & Early, 2001, p. 7). However, this continuum is not meant to be used in a strictly stepwise fashion and the various levels can overlap and be used simultaneously as required. Essentially, these intervention levels are based on the assumption that purposeful activity is the "primary treatment tool of occupational therapy" (p. 7) and that adjunctive methods and enabling activities are used as preparatory to functional activity in performance areas, rather than the aim of remediating problems in the performance components being an end in itself. As they stated, "exclusive use of such preparatory methods out of context of the patient's occupational performance is not considered OT" (p. 7).

The first level of intervention is *adjunctive methods*. These are "procedures that prepare the patient for occupational performance but are preliminary to the use of purposeful activity" (p. 7). These methods generally focus on remediating performance components or maintaining structural integrity of body parts to prevent problems that could interfere with their potential use. They include methods such as "exercise, facilitation and inhibition techniques, positioning, sensory stimulation, selected physical agent modalities, and provision of devices such as braces and splints" (p. 7). Pedretti and Early (2001) emphasized that occupational therapists using these methods need to plan for progression to the subsequent intervention levels to ensure that adjunctive methods remain preparatory to purposeful activity.

The second level is *enabling activities*. This level involves the use of activities that might not be considered purposeful. Interventions at this level often involve simulation tasks, examples of which include "sanding boards, skate boards, stacking cones or blocks, practice boards for mastery of clothing fasteners and hardware, driving simulators, work simulators, and table-top activities such as form boards for training in perceptual-motor skills" (Pedretti & Early, 2001, p. 7). These are often used when the requirements of purposeful activities are beyond the capabilities of patients. Essentially they represent graded activities that might enable patients to engage in activities for remediation and experience success, when purposeful activities would not be likely to result in this level of success. However, similar to adjunct methods, they need to be regarded as preparatory to purposeful activity. The primary goal of the first two levels of intervention is the remediation of performance components.

Pedretti and Early (2001) also included the use of equipment in this level. They listed equipment such as "wheelchairs, ambulatory aids, special clothing, communication devices, environmental control systems, and other assistive devices" (p. 7) as interventions at this level. It appears that their reason for including these devices here (rather than as environmental adaptations) could relate to purposeful activity being the main type of intervention proposed. As devices and equipment cannot be categorized as purposeful activity, they are probably conceptualized as tools for enabling performance, as are enabling activities. This approach appears to differ from some of the models presented in the following chapter, which present the environment as one of three primary intervention categories (i.e. person, environment, occupation).

The third intervention level is *purposeful activity*. Pedretti and Early (2001) emphasized that purposeful activity has always been at the core of occupational therapy. They defined purposeful activity as "activities that have an inherent or autonomous goal and are relevant and meaningful to the patient" (p. 8). It is the goal, relevance and meaningfulness to the patient that distinguishes this level from the second level, in which the activities chosen might have a goal that is meaningful to the occupational therapist but might not be evident to or valued by the client. The model assumes that activities become meaningful and purposeful to an individual because that individual needs them for functioning independently in their performance areas. Therefore, it is their contribution to the performance areas that makes activities purposeful.

At this level of intervention, purposeful activity is used for the purpose of "assessing and remediating deficits in the performance areas" (Pedretti & Early, 2001, p. 8). Thus, the focus is shifted to performance areas – compared with centring on performance components at the first two levels. Examples of the activities used are "feeding, hygiene, dressing, mobility, communication, arts, crafts, games, sports, work, and educational activities" (p. 8) and these could be conducted in the patient's home, a community agency, or a healthcare facility.

The final level of intervention refers to *occupations*. This is the highest stage in the treatment continuum and involves engaging "the patient in natural occupations in his or her living environment and in the community. The patient performs appropriate tasks of ADL, work and productive activities, and play and leisure to his or her maximum level of independence." (p. 9.) Because the core of this level is maximum independence and these activities are performed in their natural environments, active involvement in "scheduled OT" (p. 9) decreases to the point where it terminates and the individual "resumes and effectively performs valued occupational roles" (p. 9). The focus of this level of intervention moves to the performance of occupational roles within their natural context.

Pedretti and Early (2001) identified two "intervention approaches" (p. 10) that are valuable to use in conjunction with the OP model in the area of physical dysfunction. These are the biomechanical and motor control models. Each of these models provides principles for the treatment of movement problems caused by different processes. The biomechanical model "applies the mechanical principles of kinetics and kinematics to the movement of the human body. These mechanical principles deal with the way that forces acting on the body affect movement and equilibrium." (p. 10.) The biomechanical model guides the assessment and restoration of range of motion, muscle strength and endurance (muscular and cardiovascular) and the prevention and reduction of deformity. The biomechanical model is used for individuals with sensorimotor problems resulting from "motor unit or orthopaedic disorders but whose central nervous system (CNS) is intact" (p. 10). Common intervention methods include "joint measurement, muscle strength testing, kinetic activity, therapeutic exercise, and orthotics" (p. 10) and many of the common interventions from the first two levels (adjunctive methods and enabling activities) derive from the biomechanical model.

Second is the motor control model, which addresses CNS problems. Pedretti and Early (2001) identified four approaches within this model. These were the Rood and Brunnstrom approaches to movement therapy, Knott and Voss's proprioceptive neuromuscular facilitation, and Bobath's neurodevelopmental treatment. More recent publications of texts on rehabilitation for CNS problems demonstrate that the specific models used for addressing these types of problems have changed as knowledge has developed in this area. Readers are referred to more recent publications for the current approaches in this area.

These two treatment approaches (called frames of reference by other authors) are utilized in combination with the OP model to address problems in the sensorimotor performance components. Occupational therapists typically combine the OP model with other treatment approaches to provide details of interventions for other performance components. For example, they might use a cognitive-behavioural approach to understand interventions for psychosocial problems.

## HISTORICAL DESCRIPTION OF MODEL'S DEVELOPMENT

Despite the model being now somewhat dated, and no longer formally published, we have presented the OP model here because it is, arguably, the model that has influenced most pervasively the thinking of many practising occupational therapists throughout the world. This applies particularly to the area of physical dysfunction, but also more broadly.

The OP model reflected the official stance of the American Occupational Therapy Association and was influenced by their documents produced from the early 1970s. In 1996, Pedretti provided a detailed description of the history of the development of the OP model. She commenced by stating:

> *In 1973 the American Occupational Therapy Association (AOTA) published* The Roles and Functions of Occupational Therapy Personnel. *This publication referred to occupational performance as a frame of reference that included three performance skills, later named performance areas, and five performance components, later combined to become the three used in the later versions of the OP model. The purpose was to describe the areas of expertise of occupational therapists and the domains of concern within the profession. (p. 5)*

In this history, she discussed various publications throughout the 1970s and early 1980s as documents that contributed to an understanding of occupational performance. She also cited the three editions of the AOTA publication outlining recommendations for uniform reporting of occupational therapy services (which were primarily centred on hospital-based services) as documents that "defined the terminology in the occupational performance frame of reference" (p. 5). In summarizing its development, she wrote:

> *Thus, the concept of the Occupational Performance model was developed from a series of task forces and committees of the AOTA. It was generated from professional conceptualizations of practice and originally described as a frame of reference for practice and for curriculum design in education. (p. 5)*

Evident with the OP model is the influence of both the mechanistic paradigm and the beginning of the renaissance of occupation (both discussed in the introduction to this book – see Table I.1). In line with this renaissance of occupation, a change in the discourse of occupational therapy has occurred since the latter part of the twentieth century, with the term *occupation* becoming used pervasively. The sixth edition of *Occupational Therapy: Practice Skills for Physical Dysfunction* (McHugh Pendleton & Schultz-Krohn, 2006) reflects this shift towards occupation within the profession by presenting the Occupational Therapy Practice Framework (OTPF) as representing the official position of the AOTA (rather than the OP model like the previous editions). The OTPF has also been developed with the World Health Organization's International Classification of Functioning, Disability and Health (ICF) in mind, and its relationship to the ICF is emphasized in the sixth edition. This emphasis on the ICF demonstrates the shift that has also occurred in the broader healthcare environment, in which the focus has moved away from bodily impairments alone (a biomedical approach), to activity and participation (both biopsycho-social and socioecological approaches). This movement is more aligned with the current paradigm of occupation in occupational therapy.

## OCCUPATIONAL THERAPY PRACTICE FRAMEWORK (OTPF)

The OTPF reflects the current movement towards occupation as occupational therapy's core concern. However, the influence of the OP model on this frame-work is apparent. The concepts of performance areas, performance compo-nents and context are evident within this practice framework, albeit relabelled and incorporated into more detailed and additional categories. The way that the categories of the OTPF relate to the International Classification of Function (ICF) is also made explicit in the OTPF document. The OTPF has been pub-lished in two editions – 2002 and 2008. The edition used in this chapter is from 2008 and this includes a summary of the changes made to the first edition in developing the second edition. That summary is provided on pages 665–667 of the second edition (AOTA, 2008).

The OTPF aims to make explicit both the *domain* and *process* of occupa-tional therapy. According to McHugh Pendleton and Schultz-Krohn (2006), "the domain describes the scope of practice or answers the question: 'What does an occupational therapist do?' The process describes the methods of pro-viding occupational therapy services or answers the question: 'How does an occupational therapist provide occupational therapy services?' (p. 10).

## DOMAIN

The OTPF domain is divided into the following six categories: areas of occu-pation, client factors, activity demands, performance skills, performance patterns, and context and environment. The influence of the OP model is particularly evident within the first category, *areas of occupation*. This cat-egory includes activities of daily living (ADL) (also called personal or basic ADL, i.e. PADL and BADL, respectively), instrumental activities of daily living (IADL), rest and sleep, education, work, play, leisure and social par-ticipation. The OTPF emphasizes that particular occupations can only be categorized in terms of their meaning and purpose for an individual. For example, laundry might be categorized as work for one person and IADL for another.

*Client factors* are "specific abilities, characteristics, or beliefs that reside within the client and may affect performance in areas of occupation" (AOTA, 2008, p. 630). As clients of occupational therapy services could be individu-als, organizations or populations, this category is conceptualized as relevant to all three potential client groups. For each, the relevant values and beliefs, functions and structures are considered. For the person, values, beliefs and spirituality "influence a client's motivation to engage in occupations and give his or her life meaning" (p. 633).

Using terminology consistent with the ICF, *client factors* include body functions and body structures. Quoting from a WHO publication, body functions are defined as the physiological functions of body systems (including psychological functions) and body structures refer to the anatomical parts of the body such as organs, limbs and their components. For organizations, values and beliefs might be encapsulated in vision and other value statements and codes of ethics. Functions include the processes that an organization uses for its planning, organizing and operationalizing its core functions and vision. Structures relate to the way the organization is structured including departments and their relationships, leadership and management structures, performance measures, etc. For populations, values and beliefs can include "emotional, purposive, and traditional perspectives"; functions include "economic, political, social and cultural capital" and structures "may include constituents such as those with similar genetics, sexual orientation, and health-related conditions" (AOTA, 2008, p. 634).

*Activity demands* "refer to the specific features of an activity that influence the type and amount of effort required to perform the activity" (AOTA, 2008, p. 634). A core skill of occupational therapists is the analysis of activities and occupations. They use this analysis to determine the capacities required for an individual to perform these activities within particular contexts. The specific constellation of demands of performing an activity or occupation provides enormous potential for altering activity demands to enable engagement in occupation. A change in one component of the activity or the context in which it is performed changes the total demands of the activity or occupation.

*Performance skills* have the closest relationship to performance components in the OP model. Performance skills are "the abilities clients demonstrate in the actions they perform" (AOTA, 2008, p. 639). The OTPF uses the following six interrelated categories for performance skills: motor and praxis skills, sensory-perceptual skills, emotional regulation skills, cognitive skills and communication and social skills (which have similarities to the original five categories of performance components). The OTPF distinguishes between body functions and performance skills in that body functions are capacities that "reside within the body" (p. 639) whereas performance skills are those abilities that can be demonstrated. Two of the examples that were given in the OTPF document of observable nature of performance skills are as follows: "praxis skills can be observed through client actions such as imitating, sequencing, and constructing; cognitive skills can be observed as the client demonstrates organization, time management, and safety" (p. 639). In further explicating the difference, the OTPF states "numerous body functions underlie each performance skill" (p. 639).

*Performance patterns* include the "habits, routines, roles, and rituals" (p. 641) that people use when engaging in activities and occupations. All four can facilitate or make difficult engagement in and performance of occupations. Habits are automatic behaviours used for engagement in occupations; routines are "established sequences of occupations or activities that provide

Occupational performance and adaptation models

a structure for daily life" (p. 641); roles are "sets of behaviour" (p. 641) that have social and personal expectations, can have implications for self-identity, and can shape choice and meaning of occupations; and rituals are "symbolic actions with spiritual, cultural, or social meaning that contribute to the client's identity and reinforce the client's values and beliefs" (p. 642). Performance patterns can develop and change over time and assist people to organize their engagement in occupations within their daily lives and over the course of their lives. The concept of performance was not a feature of the OP model, but has become embedded in occupational therapy thinking. This possibly occurred through the pervasive influence of Kielhofner's Model of Human Occupation, presented in Chapter 6, which introduced the concept habits and routines.

Occupational therapists have always acknowledged that engagement in and performance of occupations occurs with specific places, at specific times, under specific conditions. In the OTPF, the situatedness of occupational performance is considered using the category of *context and environment*. It uses the term environment to refer to the physical and social environments. The physical environment refers to the natural and built environments (including the objects within them) in which people might perform occupations and the social environment "is constructed by the presence, relationships, and expectations of persons, groups, and organizations with whom the client has contact" (AOTA, 2008, p. 642).

While the term environment is used to refer to tangible aspects of the situation within which people engage in occupation, the term context is used to acknowledge the less tangible aspects of the circumstances surrounding occupational performance that can strongly influence it. These contexts can be "cultural, personal, temporal, and virtual" (AOTA, 2008, p. 642). The OTPF provides the following definitions of these four types of context, some of which are attributed to the WHO: "*Cultural context* includes customs, beliefs, activity patterns, behaviour standards, and expectations accepted by the society of which the client is a member. *Personal context* refers to demographic features of the individual such as age, gender, socioeconomic status, and educational level that are not part of a health condition. *Temporal context* includes stages of life, time of day or year, duration, rhythm of activity, or history. *Virtual context* refers to interactions in simulated, real-time or near-time situations absent of physical contact" (pp. 642 & 646). As these definitions demonstrate, the contexts surrounding occupational performance can be internal or external to the client or, in the case of cultural context, both internal and external contexts can combine – in that culture is an external context that shapes individual values and beliefs but the individual also internalizes these (to varying extents), making them part of the internal context of occupational performance.

## PROCESS

In addition to the occupational therapy domain, the OTPF also describes the "process that outlines the way in which occupational therapy practitioners operationalize their expertise to provide services to clients" (AOTA, 2008, p. 646). While the general processes that occupational therapists use, that is, assessment/evaluation, intervention and evaluating the outcomes, are also used by other professions, the OTPF document highlights that the distinctiveness of occupational therapy lies in its work "toward the end-goal of supporting health and participation in life through engagement in occupations" (pp. 646–647). Occupational therapists are also unique in that they conceptualize occupations as both methods and outcomes. Within a collaborative relationship with the client, occupational therapists plan for interventions on the basis of jointly identified and prioritized goals.

The first part of the process is *assessment/evaluation*. Practitioners collect sufficient appropriate information to develop an understanding of what has been, needs to be, and can be done with and for the client. The OTPF identifies this stage as consisting of both the *occupational profile* and *analysis of occupational performance*. It states, "The occupational profile includes information about the client and the client's needs, problems, and concerns about performance in areas of occupation. The analysis of occupational performance focuses on collecting and interpreting information using assessment tools designed to observe, measure, and inquire about factors that support or hinder occupational performance." (AOTA, 2008, p. 649.) These two components of the assessment/evaluation stage are described in detail in the OTPF document. Occupational therapists use their clinical reasoning to combine, analyze and synthesize information gained about the client's occupational profile and occupational performance and make decisions about intervention.

*Intervention* is defined as "the skilled actions taken by occupational therapy practitioners in collaboration with the client to facilitate engagement in occupation related to health and participation" (AOTA, 2008, p. 652). In the OTPF, the intervention process is categorized into three steps, which are not necessarily followed in a linear sequence in practice. These are development of an intervention plan, implementation of the intervention, and its review. Each step in the intervention process is discussed in detail in the OTPF document.

The third part of the occupational therapy process relates to *evaluating outcomes*. The OTPF described the overall outcome of occupational therapy intervention as "supporting health and participation in life through engagement in occupation" (AOTA, 2008, p. 660). More specific outcomes are generally required to determine the degree of progress towards this more general goal that might have resulted from occupational therapy interventions. More specific outcomes might include "clients' improved performance of occupations, perceived happiness, self-efficacy, and hopefulness about their life and abilities" (pp. 660–661). Outcomes might include information about clients' subjective impressions of relevant goals or increments of progress that are measurable. The OTPF document proposed that "outcomes for populations may include health promotion, social justice, and access to services" (p. 661). The document outlined two steps in the outcomes process. The first was "Selecting types of outcomes and measures, including but not limited to occupational performance, adaptation, health and wellness, participation, prevention, self-advocacy, quality of life, and occupational justice" (p. 661). The second step was "Using outcomes to measure progress and adjust goals and interventions" (p. 661).

## SUMMARY

In this section of the chapter, we have reviewed the OP model and the OTPF. Taken together, these two theoretical frameworks represent the major threads in occupational therapy thinking in the USA. While the OP model is no longer published, its legacy appears to have remained within both occupational therapy practice in Western countries and within the OTPF, which is currently the official document of the AOTA. The OTPF has embedded within it many of the concepts of the OP model, but these have been expanded and articulated using the current language of occupation.

Because the AOTA is clear that the OTPF is not a model of practice, we have presented a memory aid for the OP model, as that model still seems to influence much current practice. In the following section, we present a memory aid for the OP model to help make explicit how it would be used in practice.

See Box 3.1.

---

**BOX 3.1  Occupational Performance (OP) model memory aid**

**Occupational roles**
What are the person's occupational roles?

**For each role**
- What purposes do they fulfil in the person's life?

- How does the person feel about these roles?

- How do these roles influence the person's self-identity and access to social and financial resources?

In which roles, if any, is the person likely to encounter problems with performance of those roles?

- Which roles are unlikely to be affected?

How is the context in which those roles are performed likely to affect, if at all, that performance?

**Performance areas**
In the following areas, what activities does the person need/want to do to fulfil his/her occupational roles?

1. Activities of daily living (ADL)

2. Work/productivity

3. Leisure/play

**Performance components**
How is the person's capacities in the following areas influencing (if at all) his/her performance of the above activities and occupational roles?

1. Sensorimotor

2. Cognitive/cognitive integration

3. Psychosocial and psychological

---

## MAJOR WORKS

American Occupational Therapy Association (AOTA), 2008. Occupational therapy practice framework: Domain and process, second ed. Am. J. Occup. Ther. 62, 625–683.

McHugh Pendleton, H., Schultz-Krohn, W., 2006. The occupational therapy practice framework and the practice of occupational therapy for people with physical disabilities. In: McHugh Pendleton, H., Schultz-Krohn, W. (Eds.), Occupational therapy: Practice skills for physical dysfunction, sixth ed. Mosby, St Louis, MI, pp. 2–16.

Pedretti, L.W., 1996. Occupational performance: A model for practice in physical dysfunction. In: Pedretti, L.W. (Ed.), Occupational therapy: Practice skills for physical dysfunction, fourth ed. Mosby, St Louis, MI, pp. 3–12.

Pedretti, L.W., Early, M.B., 2001. Occupational performance and models of practice for physical dysfunction. In: Pedretti, L.W., Early, M.B. (Eds.), Occupational therapy: practice skills for physical dysfunction, fifth ed. Mosby, St Louis, MI, pp. 3–12.

## OCCUPATIONAL PERFORMANCE MODEL (AUSTRALIA) (OPMA)

The second model we review in this chapter is the Occupational Performance Model (Australia) (Chapparo & Ranka, 1997). This model does not represent the official position of OT Australia (the Australian Association of Occupational Therapy) in the way that the OP model represents the official position of the AOTA. Nor was it adopted by the majority of occupational therapists practising in Australia (its use was strongest in New South Wales, the Australian state in which it was developed). However, we have included this model in this book as it provides an excellent example of the influence of a biopsychosocial model of health on occupational therapy conceptual models.

### MAIN CONCEPTS AND DEFINITIONS OF TERMS

As the name suggests, the Occupational Performance Model (Australia) (OPMA) is a model that focuses on occupational performance as its central concept. It is structured in a similar way to the American OP model through *levels* of occupational performance. The OPMA addresses occupational performance on three mutually influencing levels – occupational roles, occupational performance areas and occupational performance components – as well as a fourth level that identifies three *core elements* of occupational performance: body, mind and spirit. It also includes more explicit attention to the environment than the OP model, through the concepts of space and time as factors that influence occupational performance. While the overall structure of the OPMA is similar to the OP model, particularly in its use of occupational performance areas and components, the differences in the OPMA are more consistent with other models developed or updated around a similar time (the 1990s). The trends that are evident in models at the time were towards: (1) a more integrated view of the environment and its influence on occupational performance; (2) an increased focus on and use of the term occupation (rather than activity); and (3) a biopsychosocial understanding of the person as consisting of subjective perceptions and experiences as well as body structures and functions. While the OPMA could have been included in Chapter 4 because of its extensive focus on the environment, we have included it here to emphasize the difference between the largely biomedical approach embedded in the OP model and the biopsychosocial approach of the OPMA.

Figure 3.2 provides a diagram of the OPMA. The influence of the AOTA OP model on the OPMA is evident in the structure of this diagram, in that, performance areas and performance components are presented as two different but interconnected levels in a central position in the diagram. These two concepts are central to the way that occupational performance has been conceptualized in Western countries.

However, the two models differ with regard to the detail with which they attend to the broader context on occupational performance. The diagram of the American OP model provides extensive detail about performance areas and components, represented visually as the central features of the model that contribute to an understanding of occupational performance, while the environment is placed off to one side and is given little detail. In contrast, and consistent with other occupational therapy models of practice in the 1990s, the OPMA diagram represents the environment as surrounding the person and categorizes it into four components – sensory, social, cultural and physical environments. In addition, it also shows that space and time influence occupational performance.

The OPMA diagram shows component parts of the model that are considered to be interconnected. This interconnectedness is represented in the diagram by multiple arrows. The interconnectedness is also evident in the definitions of various components and constructs, which frequently make reference to other components and constructs in their definitions.

Many models at this time conceptualized the person and environment as intimately connected. Central to the OPMA is a relationship among person, environment and occupational performance. As Chapparo and Ranka (1997)

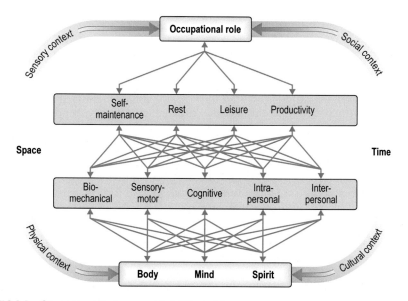

FIG 3.2 Occupational Performance Model (Australia). From http://occupationalperformance.com; created by and reprinted with kind permission of Christine Chapparro and Judy Ranka.

stated, "the primary focus of this model is the lifelong person-environment relationship and its activation through occupation" (p. 3). Evident within this quote is the assumption that occupation forms the conduit between person and occupation. As discussed in the introduction to this book, this is one of the two major ways that occupational therapists conceptualize a relationship among person, environment and occupation. A range of different models presented in this book are based on this assumed relationship between person and environment and the idea that this relationship is enabled through occupation.

The inter relatedness of person and environment is evident in the OPMA in the way the term environment is used. Rather than labelling person and environment separately, it refers to *internal and external environments* (i.e. what would often be called 'person' in other models is conceptualized here as the internal environment). With reference to the diagram, the internal environment is placed as a central column consisting of four levels – occupational performance role, performance areas, performance components, and the core elements of body, mind and spirit. Surrounding these four levels of the internal environment is the external environment. This consists of sensory, social, cultural and physical environments. The internal and external environments intersect in the diagram at the levels of occupational role and core elements. A major aspect of the model is a conceptualization of occupational performance roles as the key point of intersection between the internal and external environments.

## THE INTERNAL ENVIRONMENT

The internal environment occupies the central column of the OPMA diagram. The top level of occupational roles is the point at which the internal and external environments connect. The other three levels provide the details about the components of occupational performance.

### OCCUPATIONAL ROLES: WHERE THE INTERNAL AND EXTERNAL ENVIRONMENTS CONNECT

While the internal environment comprises occupational roles, performance areas, performance components and the core elements of body, mind and spirit, the performance of *occupational roles* is the central focus of this model. From the perspective of the OPMA, every type of intervention that occupational therapists use should be done for the purpose of facilitating the performance of occupational roles. Any interventions used by occupational therapists that target occupational performance areas and components are only used because they are expected to influence the performance of occupational roles through these other levels. (This is similar to the emphasis placed in the OTPF, described earlier.) Chapparo and Ranka (1997) defined occupational performance roles as "patterns of occupational behaviour composed of configurations of self-maintenance, productivity, leisure and rest occupations. Occupational performance roles are determined by individual person-environment-performance relationships. They are established through need and/or choice and are modified with age, ability, experience, circumstance and time" (p. 6).

This definition emphasizes four important aspects of occupational roles in the model: (1) the degree to which occupational roles are influenced by both the individual performing the roles and social expectations of role performance; (2) the importance of the broader context in determining the need for and/ choice of engagement in occupational roles; (3) the changing nature of occupational roles over time and with changing abilities, circumstances and experiences and; (4) the interconnectedness of occupational roles and occupational performance areas (and, flowing on from this, performance components).

First, the occupational roles of any particular person are configured uniquely depending on both the person's interpretation of what is required and the expectations of others (both society and significant individuals). As evident in the diagram, it is at the level of occupational roles that the internal and external environments intersect. Consequently, in conceptualizing occupational roles, the OPMA emphasizes the interaction between the person (internal environment) and the external environment in shaping those roles. As Chapparo and Ranka (1997) stated, "within the boundaries of each role acquired throughout life, expectations of performance of role related tasks are formed by both socio-cultural factors in the external environment as well as the person who becomes the role performer" (p. 4).

Definitions of roles often emphasize the social expectations associated with roles. For instance, Chapparo and Ranka used Christiansen and Baum's 1991 definition of roles, stating that a role comprises "a set of behaviours that have some socially agreed upon functions and for which there is an accepted code of norms" (p. 4). Chapparo and Ranka then commented that occupational performance roles are "those roles that constitute the bulk of daily function and routines" (p. 4). A person's role perception is dependent upon both the social expectation associated with that role and the person's own perception of the value of the role in his or her life and what he or she should or needs to do to fulfil it. The emphasis the OPMA places on the mutual influence between social and individual expectations and interpretations differentiates this model from others that conceptualize occupation as the medium through which person and occupation are connected. Whereas some other models conceptualize occupation as the vehicle through which individuals obtain mastery over the environment, the relationship between person and environment is not understood as the person *acting on* the environment through occupation. Instead, social roles encapsulate a two-way influence.

Second, the definition refers to occupational roles being established through need and/or choice. This assertion encapsulates the notion that occupational roles can fulfil a number of purposes in people's lives. Their position at the intersection between the internal and external environments emphasizes that these needs and choices are influenced by both environments. For example, a person might perceive the need to engage in a particular occupational role in a particular way in order to meet a social demand (social expectations). However, fulfilling this role might also affect how that person thinks about him- or herself (self-identity) and influence the capacities, skills and interests that the person develops. If the person's role performance is evaluated positively by both the external and internal environments, the person is likely to enjoy and pursue that role and it might become increasingly self-defining. In contrast, if the person feels that he or she has no choice but to perform that role, he or she might see it as a duty or essential for survival (or some other social purpose) rather than something to look forward to or that is self-defining. In either case, the person might or might not choose or determine the need to enhance their skills and employ them in fulfilling that role. Chapparo and Ranka (1997) also made the point that "individual choice is alien to a number of social groups whose sociocultural identity is collective" (p. 5).

Third, the OPMA proposes that a person's occupational roles change with age, ability, experience and circumstance. While a person is likely to fulfil multiple roles simultaneously, these roles and their combinations will change as the internal and external environments change. Internal environments change as people age, their capacities, skills and interests wax and wane, and their experiences and expectations of and hopes for life change. External environments change as people come and go, as the physical environments in which people perform occupational roles alter and vary, and as societies, organizations and institutions change. As the internal and external environments change, the demands placed on a person and his or her preferences, abilities and perceptions of choice combine to influence people's roles and their performance of those roles.

Fourth, in the OPMA, attention is given to performance areas and performance components in order to understand and facilitate occupational performance of roles. In this model, the central purpose of occupational therapy, a profession that often claims to promote health and well-being through occupation, is the facilitation of performance of occupational roles. Chapparo and Ranka (1997) explained the association between health and performance of occupational roles by stating, "Health is not the absence of disease, rather, it is competence and satisfaction in the performance of occupational roles, routines and tasks" (p. 2).

Chapparo and Ranka proposed that occupational performance roles have three dimensions – *knowing*, *doing* and *being* – which can contribute to occupational role performance to different degrees, depending on the abilities of the person and the demands of the role. They defined the knowing element as "having an intuitive or concrete understanding of desired or expected occupational performance roles" (p. 5). In a sense, it is about knowing what is required of you. The doing element refers to the process of carrying out occupational performance roles. Thus, it is not enough to know what is required but one also needs to be able to do what is required. The being element is described as a "fulfilment or satisfaction component of occupational performance roles" (p. 5). Because the internal and external environments are bound closely, the process of knowing about and performing occupational roles also has an effect on how the person feels and thinks about him- or herself.

## OCCUPATIONAL PERFORMANCE AREAS AND COMPONENTS AND THE CORE ELEMENTS

A primary skill of occupational therapists is being able to understand and analyze the performance of occupational roles. In the OPMA, occupational role is at the top of four levels at which occupational performance can be analyzed. The three levels below it in the diagram are all part of the internal environment. These additional levels are occupational performance areas, occupational performance components and core elements of occupational performance, which are required for the performance of social roles.

The first level is *occupational performance areas*. The definition of occupational roles provided in the OPMA makes reference to "patterns of occupational behaviour composed of configurations of self-maintenance, productivity, leisure and rest occupations" (p. 6). As with the OP model, the OPMA uses the categories of performance areas to group occupations that contribute to occupational roles. However, in identifying performance areas, the OPMA emphasizes that the process of classifying particular occupations is idiosyncratic and should be done by the performer. The performance areas into which any individual might classify particular occupations can also change over time, age, circumstance and ability.

The OPMA adds rest occupations to self-maintenance, productivity and leisure, the last three areas being traditionally used in occupational therapy discourse and aligning with the main occupational performance areas in the OP model. Rest occupations were defined as "the purposeful pursuit of non-activity" (p. 6) and include sleep and the various activities undertaken for the purpose of relaxation. Chapparo and Ranka justified the inclusion of this performance area as a separate category to self-maintenance occupations by stating that "there are socio-cultural, daily and life span reasons for the degree to which people are, or wish to be, passive and contemplative rather than active and productive" (pp. 6–7). This rationale acknowledges the way the external environment can influence a person's occupational behaviour. In contrast, categorizing rest as self-maintenance activities would be emphasizing the internal moderation aspects of the behaviour, rather than the need or choice to respond to external demands and influences.

The performance areas are a way of categorizing occupations into groups. However, OPMA further categorizes occupations into types of activity. The model does not use the term 'activity' because the authors argued that the "meanings attributed to the underlying construct [activity] have become so broad and flexible that it has lost its power to 1) describe elements of occupations and performance at varying levels, and 2) direct and influence the focus of occupational therapy intervention" (p. 7). Consequently, the model divides occupations into the subcategories of subtasks, tasks and routines. Subtasks are "steps or single units of the total task and are stated in terms of observable behaviour" and tasks are "sequences of subtasks that are ordered from the first performed to the last performed to accomplish a specific purpose" (p. 7). Chapparo and Ranka (1997) gave the example of the task of drinking, which can be divided into subtasks such as locating, reaching for, grasping and lifting the drinking vessel. These subtasks are performed in an orderly sequence in order to accomplish the task of drinking. Routines constitute the third subcategory and are "sequences of tasks that begin in response to an internal or an external cue and end with the achievement of the identified critical function" (p. 8). Routines are usually established to support the performance of occupations within the performance areas (i.e. self-maintenance, productivity, leisure and rest).

In the OPMA, all three subcategories of occupations are considered able to be classified according to structure and time. However, routines are discussed in more detail than tasks and subtasks in relation to both constructs. Chapparo and Ranka (1997) explained that routines have either *fixed or flexible structures* and *regular or intermittent temporal patterns*. Some routines have a fixed structure, in which they might show little deviation from established sequences of tasks and subtasks. Other routines can be undertaken using a greater variation in its components. Routines can also be fixed or intermittent in their temporal patterns. Regular routines can often become habitual "whereby the routine of well-practiced sequences of tasks can be performed without thinking" (p. 8). Intermittent routines do not have the same regularity but can be just as critical to the performance of occupations. The temporal aspects of routines, tasks and subtasks also vary with age, circumstance and ability.

The second level that contributes to the performance of occupational roles is *performance components*. Chapparo and Ranka (1997) stated, "accomplishment of routines and tasks in the occupational performance areas is predicated on the ability to sustain efficient physical, psychological and social function" (pp. 9–10). The OPMA presents a complicated view of performance components in that it conceptualizes this level as "forming both the component attributes of the performer as well as the components of the occupational tasks" (p. 10). As the authors explained, "there are physical, sensory-motor, cognitive and psychosocial dimensions to any task performed. These dimensions mirror and prompt a person's various physical, sensory-motor, cognitive and psychosocial operations which are used to engage in task performance" (p. 10). Therefore, for each of the five performance components that it addresses – biomechanical, sensory-motor, cognitive, intrapersonal, interpersonal – it presents that component from the perspective of the performer and pertaining to the aspects of the task. Table 3.2 provides the details of each of these perspectives.

The final internal level comprises the interaction of the *core elements* of body, mind and spirit. Chapparo and Ranka (1997) quoted Adolf Meyer, "our body is not merely so many pounds of flesh and bone figuring as a machine, with an abstract mind or soul added to it" (pp. 11–12). Meyer's comments were made in the context of the time when the biomedical model prevailed and a focus on the body was widespread. By making explicit the importance of body, mind and spirit (not just the body), the OPMA affirmed its position within a biopsychosocial perspective.

The body element comprises "all of the tangible physical elements of human structure"; the mind element is defined as "the core of our conscious and unconscious intellect which forms the basis of our ability to understand and reason", and the spiritual element "is defined loosely as that aspect of humans which seeks a sense of harmony within self and between self, nature, others and in some cases an ultimate other; seeks an existing mystery to life; inner conviction; hope and meaning" (Chapparo & Ranka 1997, pp. 12–13). Chapparo and Ranka summed up the relationship between these different core elements of occupational performance by stating:

> Together the body, mind, and spirit form the human body, the human brain, the human mind, the human consciousness of self and the human awareness of the universe. Relative to occupational performance, the body-mind-spirit core element of this model translates into the 'doing-knowing-being' dimensions of performance. These doing-knowing-being dimensions are fundamental to all occupational performance roles, routines, tasks and subtasks and components of occupational performance. (p. 13)

| Performance component | Perspective of the performer during task performance | Aspects of the task |
|---|---|---|
| Biomechanical | Operation of and interaction between physical structures of the body, e.g. range of motion | Biomechanical attributes of the task, e.g. size, weight |
| Sensory-motor | Operation of and interaction between sensory input and motor responses of the body, e.g. regulation of muscle activity | Sensory aspects of the task, e.g. colour, texture |
| Cognitive | Operation of and interaction between mental processes, e.g. thinking, perceiving, judging | Cognitive dimensions of the task – usually determined by its symbolic and operational complexity |
| Intrapersonal | Operation of and interaction between internal psychological processes, e.g. emotions, mood, affect, rationality | Intrapersonal attributes that can be stimulated by the tasks and are required for effective task performance, e.g. valuing, satisfaction, motivation |
| Interpersonal | The continuing and changing interaction between a person and others. . . that contributes to the development of the individual as a participant in society, e.g. relationships in partnerships, families, communities requiring sharing, cooperation, empathy | The nature and degree of interpersonal interaction required for effective task performance |

Table 3.2 *Component attributes of the performer and components of occupational tasks*

## THE EXTERNAL ENVIRONMENT

Surrounding the internal environment and linked to it, especially through occupational roles, is the external environment. In OPMA, the external environment is conceptualized as having four dimensions – sensory, physical, social and cultural – that are all interconnected. All of these external factors influence occupational roles and their performance.

The *physical environment* refers to "the natural and constructed surroundings of a person" (p. 15). This forms the physical boundaries within which occupational performance takes place. The demands of the physical environment shape occupational performance by determining the skills and abilities required to perform particular routines, tasks and subtasks in a particular location and/or position. Chapparo and Ranka (1997) also proposed that the physical environment is shaped by the sociocultural environment and provided the example of the configuration of a large Western city being quite different to a tropical village on a Pacific island.

Chapparo and Ranka (1997) proposed that the *sensory environment* "provides the natural cues that direct occupational performance" (p. 15) and connects most closely to the sensory and cognitive performance components.

The *cultural environment* "is composed of systems of values, beliefs, ideals and customs which are learned and communicated to contribute to the behavioural boundaries of a person or group of people" (p. 15). Cultural expectations of how people should behave and what they should do influence which occupational roles people need or choose to fulfil, how they formulate those roles, and how they see and feel about themselves (self-identity). In the OPMA, *social environment* is defined as "an organized structure created by the patterns of relationships between people who function in a group which in turn contributes to establishing the boundaries of behaviour" (p. 15).

The way that the external environment is discussed demonstrates the degree to which the OPMA emphasizes the influence of the environment on human behaviour. As the authors stated, "many occupational performance roles, routines, tasks and subtasks are performed specifically in response to external demands leading to constant adaptation of occupational behaviour" (Chapparo & Ranka, 1997, p. 15). However they also presented the view that the external environment can change or be maintained as a result of occupational performance. Therefore, it is important to see the internal and external environments as mutually influencing.

## CONSTRUCTS OF SPACE AND TIME

In the OPMA, the notions of space and time are understood to pervade occupational performance. Both concepts are discussed in terms of their physical manifestation and how they are experienced. Chapparo and Ranka (1997) referred to these notions as physical and felt space and time. The notion of *physical space* is derived from the concepts of physics and includes "our understanding about body structures, body systems, objects with which people interact and the wider physical world within which people exist and function" (p. 16). *Felt space* refers to the subjective experience of space. This might include "the meaning [people] attribute to it, the way they use it and their interactions within it" (p. 16). The model emphasizes that the way physical space is experienced (felt) during occupational performance pervades all of the internal levels of occupational performance. For example, the size and shape of physical objects will activate receptors and responses at the performance component level, which will be interpreted at the level of the body–mind–spirit core elements and all of this subjective experience will contribute to the performance of occupations and occupational roles.

As with space, time is discussed in terms of physical and felt time. *Physical time* relates to the laws of physics and can be seen in processes like the measurement of time and the regular movement of the sun and moon. Chapparo and Ranka (1997) defined and explained *felt time* as follows: "Felt time is a person's understanding of time based on the meaning that is attributed to it. . . felt time involves highly personal abstractions of time that have representation at all levels of the model. It is an experiential abstraction that is being constantly changed and modified by experience." (p. 18.) Both physical and felt time influence occupational performance. For example, physical time is important when recording muscle contraction and response times. It often shapes routines and deadlines by which tasks and subtasks need to be completed. Felt time might influence performance through phenomena such as the sense a person has of how much time is available for the occupation and whether he or she feels it can be accomplished in that time or whether it is the 'right' time for something.

## OCCUPATIONAL PERFORMANCE

The overall purpose of the OPMA is to provide a framework to address "both the nature of human occupations and occupational therapy practice" (Chapparo & Ranka, 1997, p. 1). Occupational performance is the major construct used to address these aims. Chapparo and Ranka defined occupational performance as "the ability to perceive, desire, recall, plan and carry out roles, routines, tasks and subtasks for the purpose of self-maintenance, productivity, leisure and rest in response to demands of the internal and/or external environment" (p. 4).

This definition gives important cues for understanding this model and some of its unique aspects. The first part of the definition refers to perceiving and desiring and points to the inclusion of and focus on an individual's subjective experience within the model. The model acknowledges that occupational performance depends upon the individual's perceptions and experiences of the world and his or her place within it. According to the definition, occupational performance depends on the person perceiving the need to perform occupation and forming a desire to do this. The concept of occupational role helps to explain how this need and desire are created. People fulfil occupational roles in their lives through their occupational performance. Fulfilling roles is not the only reason why people perceive the need and desire for occupational performance, for example, they might just enjoy it. But roles are important influences on this process of generating need and desire, as they are often vehicles for "social involvement and productive participation" (Chapparo & Ranka, 1997, p. 4). While the agency of people in shaping their occupational roles is acknowledged, the influence of the external environment in pressing upon and influencing occupational behaviour is strongly emphasized throughout the OPMA.

Chapparo and Ranka (1997) explained that occupational roles are determined by the unique interaction between the person, environment and performance, are established through need and/or choice, and change with age, ability, experience, circumstance and time. Individuals have unique constellations of roles that create specific demands for occupational performance, depending upon their life circumstances, goals and desires. These will also change for an individual over the course of his or her lifespan and as circumstances change. Because occupational roles lie at the interface between the internal and external environment, they influence and are influenced by both. For example, the external environment will influence the degree of choice that an individual has over their occupational performance roles and an individual will take on and carry out occupational roles according to his or her interests, capabilities, needs and aspirations.

"Recall, plan and carry out" are the next elements of the definition of occupational performance. They focus our attention on the ability to perform the occupations that are desired or perceived as necessary. The model asserts that performance of occupations requires "the ability to sustain efficient physical, psychological and social function" (p. 10), pointing to the importance of performance components. Occupational therapists develop skills in breaking down occupations and tasks into their components and analyzing the capacities required to accomplish them. This part of the definition points to the cognitive requirements of recalling and planning as well as the broader range of performance components that might be required to carry out the specific occupations. Because performance components relate to both the perspective of the performer and the demands of the task, in this model, occupational analysis requires consideration of how well the personal capacities and the task demands match.

In defining occupational performance, the authors combined their definitions of both performance and occupation. The performance aspect of the definition makes explicit the processes involved in the *performing* of occupations in terms of the ability to recall, plan and carry out those things that people want and need to do. However, the final part of the definition of occupational performance focuses on occupation, pointing to what people do. Occupation was defined as, "the purposeful and meaningful engagement in roles, routines, tasks and subtasks for the purpose of self-maintenance, productivity, leisure and rest" (p. 4). This definition is concerned with *what* people do and the *purposes* these occupations serve in their lives.

This definition presents occupation as a process rather than an entity. That is, it suggests that occupation is (the process of) "purposeful and meaningful engagement" rather than the things in which people engage (which are roles, routines, tasks and subtasks). Thus, when people engage in roles and tasks for the purpose of meeting needs relating to performance areas, they are engaged in the process of occupation.

The final part of the definition reads, "in response to the internal and/or external environment" (p. 4). This part of the definition emphasizes that the roles and activities that people perform are influenced by both their own skills, abilities, interests and desires and the demands of the external environment. The assumption that both environments (internal and external) are mutually influencing is central to this model. As Chapparo and Ranka stated, "Competence and satisfaction with role performance is therefore based on internal as well as external perceptions of performance" (p. 4).

## HISTORICAL DESCRIPTION OF MODEL'S DEVELOPMENT

As with many of the practice models reviewed later in this book, the impetus for the development of the OPMA came from the need for a theoretical framework to guide the curriculum at a particular institution that trained occupational therapists. In this case it was the University of Sydney, Australia. The authors stated that development of the model was commenced in 1986 "when it became clear that existing notions of occupational performance used to structure curriculum content in the Bachelor of Applied Science in Occupational Therapy at Cumberland College of Health Sciences (now The University of Sydney) required expansion to more adequately reflect both the nature of human occupations and occupational therapy practice" (Chapparo & Ranka, 1997, p. 1).

Chapparo and Ranka (1997) explained that this school of occupational therapy was required to undergo 5-yearly curriculum reviews and that, from the mid-1970s to the mid 1990s, the curriculum had changed considerably.

They explained that the changes in this period led to "the development of a theoretical framework for the curriculum which [had] two integrated conceptual thrusts" (p. 24). These were: (1) a movement towards "problem-based, adult learning modes of education"; and (2) the use of the "conceptual notions of occupational performance and functions to organize content within the curriculum" (p. 24).

As Chapparo and Ranka stated, "the process of model building was initially stimulated by curriculum restructuring and subsequently continued by the authors to develop a model of occupational performance that was relevant to occupational therapy practice in Australia" (p. 24). They also stated that, in 1997, the OPMA model was at the stage of development where "concepts have been developed, classified and related, but not yet fully evaluated or tested" (p. 2).

The model was developed in five stages. These were:

1. 1989–1990 A review of the literature. This process led to the development of a model centred on occupational performance with two levels, presumably occupational performance areas and occupational performance components.
2. 1990–1991 "Field testing" (p. 28) of this model in the practice areas of neurology and adult rehabilitation. This led to the addition of a third level to the model, presumably occupational performance roles. The authors also added the construct of occupational performance environment, most likely conceptualized as surrounding the three levels in the model.
3. 1991–1992 Field testing the three level model in acute care, paediatrics and adult rehabilitation. This stage led to the addition of the fourth level of the model, which appears to have been the core elements of body, mind and spirit. The authors also listed "development of philosophy and assumptions" (p. 28) as an outcome of this stage.
4. 1992–1994 Field testing of the four level model with the six constructs of occupational performance, occupational performance areas, occupational performance components, occupational performance roles, occupational performance environment and core elements. This field testing was undertaken in the practice areas of adult rehabilitation, community paediatric practice, psychiatry and OT administration. This stage led to acceptance of the four level model with the addition of two further constructs, space and time.
5. 1994–1996 The final stage was described as "ongoing field testing" (p. 28) in which the constructs were consolidated and refined in practice contexts through the use of written examples provided to occupational therapists. The methods used in the field testing stages of the model development included continuing professional education workshops, the use of "intervention scenarios" (p. 34) in which videotapes of clients and case studies were used as the stimulus for practitioners to plan interventions and discuss use in their own practice. Specific tasks were used to elicit practitioners' beliefs "about human potential, health, occupations, and occupational therapy" (p. 35) when developing a "personal frame of reference for practice" (p. 35).

While a monograph was published in 1997, which included many of the papers and presentations given regarding the model, the major way that the model is made available currently is through its website. This can be found at http://www.occupationalperformance.com. A number of assessments have also been devised, based on OPMA. These include the Perceive, Recall, Plan and Perform System of Task Analysis (PRPP) and the Comparative Analyses of Performance (CAPs).

## SUMMARY

OPMA provides an excellent example of the trends that occurred in occupational therapy models of practice in the mid to late 1990s. When contrasted with the OP model, it highlights the difference between a biomedical approach to health, which emphasized the body and normative views of its function and dysfunction, and a biopsychosocial view, which takes a more holistic approach to the person and considers biological, psychological and social aspects of human health and experience. It also forms a bridge to the ecological models presented in Chapter 4, as it starts to 'blur' the boundary between person and environment, through the concepts of internal and external environment.

See Box 3.2.

---

**BOX 3.2 OPMA memory aid**

What occupational roles does the person want or need to do?

**For each role**

■ Which performance area would the person use to categorize that role?

■ What routines, tasks & subtasks are needed for that person to fulfil that role?

■ What performance components (both person's capacities and activity demands) are required for performance of these routines, tasks and subtasks?

■ What aspects, if any, of the body, mind & spirit might influence or be influenced by role performance?

■ How will the physical, sensory, social and cultural environments influence and be influenced by performance of that role?

## MAJOR WORKS

Chapparo, C., Ranka, J., 1997. OPM: Occupational Performance Model (Australia), Monograph 1. Occupational Performance Network, Castle Hill, NSW.

Chapparo, C., Ranka, J., 1996. Research development. In: Chapparo, C., Ranka, J. (Eds.), The PRPP research training manual: continuing professional education. Edition 2.0, Chapter 9. Available at http://occupationalperformance.com/Index.php?/au/home/assessments/prpp/the_perceive_recall_plan_perform_prpp_system_of_task_analysis.

OPMA website. Available at http://www.occupationalperformance.com

## OCCUPATIONAL ADAPTATION

The third model presented in this chapter is Occupational Adaptation (OA) (first published by Schkade & Schultz, 1992). This model has been included in this chapter because of its emphasis on foundational concepts in occupational therapy – occupation, adaptation and mastery – and also because it is based on normative assumptions about these concepts. Just as biomedicine is based on a normative view of the body, OA understands adaptation as a normative process. However, the OA model differs from the other models presented in this chapter, because, as its name suggests, its focus is on occupational adaptation rather than occupational performance. It distinguishes between the two concepts by conceptualizing occupational performance as a behavioural outcome and occupational adaptation as an internal process of generalization.

In the various presentations of the model, an emphasis is placed on the 'normative' nature of this OA process, meaning that occupational adaptation is a normal human process that occurs across the lifespan, rather than something that only occurs when illness, stress or disability requires adaptation. Therefore, in a number of publications, readers are encouraged to apply the model to their own lives. For example, Schkade and McClung (2001) stated, "we recommend that a therapist wishing to use this perspective in intervention should first 'try it on' with regard to his or her own life role adaptation challenges" (pp. 2–3) in order to enhance the person's understanding of the model.

### MAIN CONCEPTS AND DEFINITIONS OF TERMS

The Occupational Adaptation (OA) model aims to provide a framework for conceptualizing the process by which humans respond adaptively to their environments. The name of the model comes from combining the concepts of occupation and adaptation, which were both foundational concepts for occupational therapy. Schultz and Schkade (1997) defined adaptation as a change in one's response to the environment when encountering an occupational challenge. As they stated, "This change is implemented when the individual's customary response approaches are found inadequate for producing some degree of mastery over the challenge" (p. 474). Their definition of adaptation encompasses two important aspects: the need for a *changed response* and the idea of *mastery*.

In emphasizing the need for a changed response, Schultz (2009) stated, "Most occupational therapy is driven by the assumption that, as clients become more functional, they will be more adaptive." (p. 463.) However, Schultz and

USING OCCUPATIONAL THERAPY MODELS IN PRACTICE

Schkade (1997) stressed that function and adaptation are not the same thing and that increased function does not necessarily mean increased adaptation. They stated, "Therapists may incorrectly assume that as the patient acquires more functional skills, or begins using assistive devices, adaptation is occurring. [However], the individual's internal adaptation may remain unchanged." (p. 460.) Their definitions and discussions suggest that occupational adaptation is a process that must occur internally, within the individual.

The second concept that underpins the model is mastery. The model is based on the assumption that individuals *desire* mastery, environments *demand* it and the interaction between the two *presses* for it. This combination of ideas about mastery forms the starting point in the diagrammatic representation of the model (Figure 3.3). This diagram is presented as a temporal "freeze-frame sketch" (Schkade & Schultz, 2003, p. 183) of the process of occupational adaptation that enables its components to be analyzed in depth. However, they made the point that the process actually operates rapidly as individuals are often required to deal with multiple occupational challenges simultaneously and that the diagram only represents one "pass" through the process, which, in reality, might require more rotations.

The model contains "three overarching elements: the person, the occupational environment and their interaction" and, for each of these elements, a "constant factor" is provided (Schultz, 2009, p. 465). The three elements are represented in the diagram by three columns with the person and occupational environment on the outer edges and the interaction between the two in the centre. The diagram starts with a circle in each column outlining the

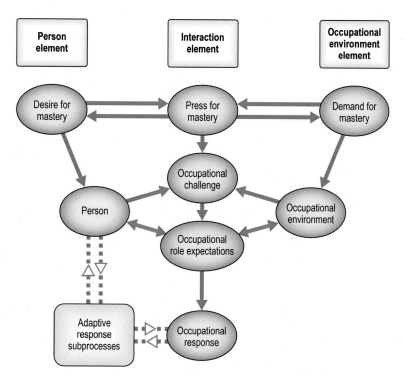

FIG 3.3   Occupational Adaptation model.

relevant constant factor (or assumption about mastery). That is, to the left of the diagram, under person, the constant factor is *desire for mastery*; on the right, under occupational environment, it is *demand for mastery*; and in the centre, under interaction, it is *press for mastery*. These concepts are presented as "dynamic, ever-changing" (p. 465) states that are mutually influencing. It is this combined desire, demand and press for mastery that provides the impetus for humans to face occupational challenges and make adaptive responses. Adaptive responses are achieved through engagement in occupation.

In explaining the person element of the model, also referred to as internal factors of the OA process, Schultz (2009) presented the *desire for mastery* over the environment as a "constant factor in the OA process" (p. 465), in that, it is always present. Drawing upon Reilly's work, she claimed that "even at a cellular level, there is constant demand for adaptation and mastery" and stated that this desire is "an innate human condition" (p. 465). The innate nature of this need is central to the model (Schkade & McClung, 2001; Schkade & Schultz, 1992, 2003; Schultz, 2009). The person is conceptualized as consisting of unique sensorimotor, cognitive and psychosocial systems, which are affected by biological, genetic and phenomenological influences and all of which are required for occupation.

In this model, the external factors that affect the person are referred to as the occupational environment. The *demand for mastery* is seen as the constant factor relating to the occupational environment. As Schultz (2009) stated, "OA theory proposes that any circumstance presents itself with at least a minimal degree of demand for mastery" (p. 465). Schkade and Schultz (2003) proposed that the mastery demanded by the environment is dependent on its physical, social and cultural features. They stated that "failure to respond with sufficient mastery produces lack of reinforcement at best and punishment at worst" (p. 187). The term occupational environment is used in the model to emphasize the link between mastery and occupation, in that, occupation is the vehicle through which people pursue mastery. Therefore, the term occupational environment is considered to represent "the overall context within which the person engages in the particular occupation and occupational role" (Schultz, 2009, p. 465).

The fact that people fulfil occupational roles is central to the process by which the environment demands mastery. Individuals' occupational roles shape how the context in which they live demands occupation of them. Schultz (2009) explained that there are three types of *occupational environments*, which she listed as work, play/leisure and self-care (readers will recognize these as the performance areas in occupational performance models). When using the model, Schkade and Schultz (2003) proposed that occupational therapists need to understand the specific demands that the occupational environment places on any particular individual in order to be able to devise interventions that are appropriate to their occupational needs.

The third element of the OA process is the interaction between the internal and external factors, or person and occupational environments. According to Schultz (2009), "The internal and external factors are continuously interacting with each other through the modality of occupation" (p. 465). The two constants associated with the person and occupational environment – desire for mastery and demand for mastery – combine to create the *press for mastery*.

In the diagrammatic representation, the interaction between the internal and external factors lies in the centre, where the OA processes are outlined. In this process, the press for mastery creates an occupational challenge. This occupational challenge, in turn, "always suggests occupational role expectations" (Schkade & Schultz, 2003, p. 191). Schultz (2009) explained the process in this way: "The *occupational role expectations* of the person and of the occupational environment intersect in response to the unique occupational challenge that the individual experiences. A demand for adaptation occurs. The person makes an internal adaptive response to the situation and then produces an *occupational response*. The *occupational response* is the outcome – the observable by-product of the adaptive response." (p. 465, italics in original.) This response might be an action or behaviour.

The OA model could be conceptualized as having two major parts to it. The first is the process, described previously, of moving from the press for mastery to an occupational response. In the diagram, this process is represented by the shaded ovals in both the central column (interaction element) and at the top on each side of the diagram – the desire for mastery and the person elements on the left and the demand for mastery and occupational environment elements on the right. The second part details the process by which individuals make adaptive responses. These are referred to as "subprocesses" (Schultz, 2009, p. 465) and are represented by the left box in the diagram. The details of the subprocesses are provided in Figure 3.4. All three subprocesses are internal to the person.

The three adaptive response processes are the Adaptive Response Generation Subprocess, the Adaptive Response Evaluation Subprocess and the Adaptive Response Integration Subprocess. These subprocesses cover generating, evaluating and integrating adaptive responses. First, the *Adaptive Response Generation Subprocess* allows the person to generate a response to the occupational challenge and its consequent occupational role expectations. The process of generating an adaptive response has two stages, called the adaptive response mechanism and the adaptation gestalt. The first stage details how the person readies him- or herself to make a response and in the second stage the person "configures his or her person systems (sensorimotor, cognitive and psychosocial) to carry out the plan" (Schultz, 2009, p. 467). Thus, the subprocess of generating a response requires both preparing for and executing that response.

Readers are referred to the various publications about the model, which provide greater details about the subprocesses. In particular, the chapter by Schkade and Schultz (2003) provides substantial detail about each of the

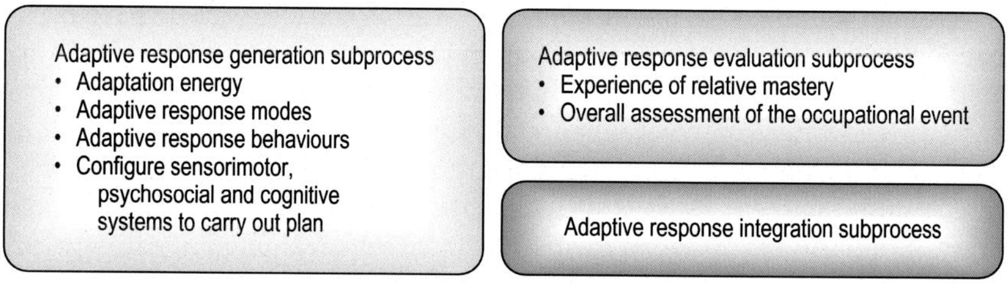

Adaptive response generation subprocess
• Adaptation energy
• Adaptive response modes
• Adaptive response behaviours
• Configure sensorimotor,
   psychosocial and cognitive
   systems to carry out plan

Adaptive response evaluation subprocess
• Experience of relative mastery
• Overall assessment of the occupational event

Adaptive response integration subprocess

FIG 3.4   Adaptive response subprocess.

elements and subprocesses of the model. For simplicity, however, only a summary is provided here. In preparing to make a response, the individual uses *adaptation energy*. For example, they might think directly about a problem or they might think about it while doing something else. Either way, the individual is investing energy into formulating an adaptive response. He or she will also need to choose "adaptive patterns or strategies that the individual has established through life experiences" (Schultz, 2009, p. 467). These could be new strategies, existing strategies or modifications of existing strategies and are referred to as *adaptive response modes*. Individuals will also choose from *adaptive response behaviours*, which are considered to be "hyperstable, hypermobile, and transactional" (p. 467). These are behaviours that are characterized, respectively, by persistence in a course of action, rapid movement between different behaviours and a combination of the previous two. Once they have used these three elements to prepare for generating a response, individuals then gather their unique sensorimotor, cognitive and psychosocial capacities and make the response.

Schultz (2009) clarified that individuals "produce an internal adaptive response to the occupational challenge" (p. 467) and that the occupational response is the product of this internal response. She then went on to explain that, "Although the adaptive response is not directly observable, it does become operationalized within the occupational response. The nature of the internal adaptive response can be gleaned readily from careful observation and analysis of the individual's approach to the task, his or her problem-solving methods, and the resulting outcomes" (p. 467).

Once the occupational response has been made, the individual needs to evaluate its quality. The process by which this is undertaken is called the *Adaptive Response Evaluation Subprocess*. Because the occupational response is a consequence of the desire, demand and press for mastery, the criterion used to assess the quality of the occupational response is *relative mastery*. This term emphasizes the fact that individuals experience mastery uniquely, relative to how well they feel their occupational response met the occupational challenge within the context of their occupational roles. The model proposes four criteria by which people evaluate their relative mastery. These are: "efficiency (use of time, energy, resources); effectiveness (the extent to which the desired goal was achieved); satisfaction to self; and satisfaction to society" (p. 467). Each criterion is evaluated as negative, positive or neutral. The same evaluation standards are used to make a judgement about the adaptiveness of the overall occupational response. Using adaptation terms, these three standards are labelled disadaptive (negative), homeostasis (neutral) and adaptive (positive).

The final subprocess is the *Adaptive Response Integration Subprocess*. An occupational response only becomes an adaptive response when it leads to the ability to generalize. This process requires memory and reflection. Positive or negative evaluation of occupational responses can lead to integration of that response. Memories of occupational responses that led to positive results can be stored in memory as strategies that could potentially be useful in the future. Similarly, occupational responses that were evaluated negatively can prompt the person to reflect upon why he or she obtained the particular outcome and what might be done differently in the future in a similar situation.

Schkade and Schultz (2003) clarified that "it is not skill mastery that produces generalization, but rather the adaptive capacity put to use… Without the adaptive capacity to anticipate outcomes, the individual is left with an array of specific skills whose applicability is specific rather than general." (p. 207.)

In summary, the three subprocesses offer an explanation of the process by which an individual generates and executes a response to an occupational challenge, evaluates it, and then generalizes from the experience. This sequence of subprocesses enables the individual to adapt to and learn from his or her experiences and, therefore, equips them more strongly to respond adaptively to future occupational challenges, resulting in occupational adaptation.

## HISTORICAL DESCRIPTION OF MODEL'S DEVELOPMENT

This model was developed by the occupational therapy faculty at Texas Woman's University in the USA as a framework upon which to build their research program and their Doctor of Philosophy in Occupational Therapy program. As Schultz (2009) explained, "One of the group's challenges was to name and frame how the program would contribute to the discipline and practice of occupational therapy". According to Schkade and Schultz (2003), the faculty decided that the focus of their research program should be the concepts of occupation and adaptation as these two concepts were "historically important and central to occupational therapy" (p. 183). Consequently, their theoretical frame of reference was labelled Occupational Adaptation. In the years from 1994 (when the Doctoral program was established) to 2007, 30 students had graduated from the program (Schultz, 2009).

It appears that the faculty have approached their research under the umbrella of occupational adaptation in different ways, with some faculty using a qualitative grounded theory methodology (Schkade & Schultz gave the examples of Spencer et al., 1998; Spencer & Davidson, 1998; Spencer et al., 1999; White, 1998), while Schkade and Schultz have become associated with the model that has become known as 'Occupational Adaptation' because they were "asked to develop the group's conceptualization of occupational adaptation into the perspective that would be the core of the doctoral program" (Schultz, 2009, p. 463). Anne Henderson, Lela Llorens and Kathlyn Reed were asked to provide ongoing consultation into this process. According to Schultz (2009), Occupational Adaptation was introduced as a frame of reference in 1992 and in 2003 as an "overarching theory for occupational therapy practice and research" (p. 463).

Emphasizing the significance of the historical inheritance of these ideas upon which Occupational Adaptation is based, Schultz (2009) stated that "the intellectual heritage of this theory dates back to the writings of William Dunton (1913) and Adolf Meyer (1922)" (p. 463). The other, more recent, occupational therapy writer whose work reportedly influenced the model was Mary Reilly. Her concept of the importance of mastery to the health and well-being of humans is a central concept within the model.

Also emphasizing the occupational therapy heritage of the model, Schkade and Schultz (1992) listed four theories that they claimed had "similarity with the proposed construct of occupational adaptation" (p. 830). These were Gilfoyle, Grady and Moore's spatiotemporal adaptation (1990), a model of adaptation through occupation by Reed (1984), Kielhofner's Model of Human Occupation (1985) and a model of occupation by Nelson (1988). However, they did not outline what aspects of these models had similarities with the OA model and how.

The OA model has not changed very much (compared to some other models reviewed in this book) since its early presentations in 1992. Publications have been authored by various combinations of Schkade and Schultz and other co-authors. The main process that the various publications have followed is to clarify some of the concepts, rather than to develop the model. In particular, the book by Schkade and McClung (2001) focused particularly on applying the model in practice. Other publications have provided briefer overviews of the model (e.g. Schultz, 2009).

## SUMMARY

Unlike many of the other models of practice presented in this book, OA focuses on occupational adaptation rather than occupational performance. It distinguishes between occupational performance as a behavioural outcome that may or may not result in occupational adaptation, which is seen as an internal process. The model assumes that people's desire for mastery interacts with the environment's demand for mastery, creating a press for mastery. This press, in turn, creates an occupational challenge. People can respond to this challenge adaptively using subprocesses that allow them to generate a response, evaluate that response and then integrate the response. Integrating the response allows the person to generalize from that particular instance. Depending upon how the response has been evaluated, the person may choose to use that response again or not in similar situations. This process of occupational adaptation is considered to operate rapidly and repeatedly as people usually deal with multiple occupational challenges simultaneously.

See Box 3.3.

---

**BOX 3.3** Occupational Adaptation memory aid

What occupational challenges is this person currently facing?

**For each role**
- How is this person's desire for mastery contributing to these?

- How is the environment's demand for mastery contributing to these?

- How are the desire and demand for mastery combining to generate a press for mastery that is creating these occupational challenges?

What occupational role expectations will be affected by these occupational challenges and how?

**For each role**
- Could these current role expectations be changed so they can be fulfilled successfully? If so, how (changes to person and/or environment)?

Occupational responses

- What occupational responses are required to enable the person to fulfil his/her role expectations in the relevant environment?

- How well is the person generating, evaluating and integrating these occupational responses? If needed, what could be done to improve this process?

---

## MAJOR WORKS

Schkade, J.K., McClung, M., 2001. Occupational Adaptation in practice: Concepts and cases. Slack, Thorofare, NJ.

Schkade, J.K., Schultz, S., 1992. Occupational Adaptation: Toward a holistic approach to contemporary practice, Part 1. Am. J. Occup. Ther. 46, 829–837.

Schkade, J.K., Schultz, S., 2003. Occupational Adaptation. In: Kramer, P., Hinosa, J., Royeen, C. (Eds.), Perspectives in human occupation. Lippincott Williams & Wilkins, Philadelphia, PA, pp. 181–221.

Schultz, S., 2009. Theory of Occupational Adaptation. In: Crepeau, E.B., Cohn, E.S., Boyt Schell, B.A. (Eds.), Willard & Spackman's occupational therapy, eleventh ed. Lippincott Williams & Wilkins, Philadelphia, PA, pp. 462–475.

Schultz, S., Schkade, J.K., 1992. Occupational Adaptation: Toward a holistic approach to contemporary practice, Part 2. Am. J. Occup. Ther. 46, 917–926.

Schultz, S., Schkade, J.K., 1997. Adaptation. In: Christiansen, C., Baum, C. (Eds.), Occupational therapy: Enabling function and well-being, second ed. Slack, Thorofare, NJ, pp. 458–481.

## CONCLUSION

In this chapter we reviewed three occupational therapy models of practice. These were the AOTA OP model, the OPMA and OA. The first two models come from the tradition of occupational therapy theory that detailed the internal capacities of the person that affect their occupational performance. These were originally referred to as *performance components*, a term that has persisted within occupational therapy thought and discourse. One of the major differences between the two models is the biopsychosocial emphasis inherent within the OPMA.

A second major concept in occupational therapy discourse is adaptation to and mastery of the environment. The concepts of occupation and adaptation are central to the Occupational Adaptation model. Whereas the occupational performance models focus on occupational performance, the Occupational Adaptation model distinguishes between the performance of occupation and adaptation to the environment.

In Chapter 4, three models focusing on environment as particularly important are presented. These are the Person-Environment-Occupation-Performance (PEOP) model, the Person-Environment-Occupation (PEO) model and the Ecology of Human Performance (EHP). While the environment is an important component of the three models of practice presented in this chapter, the last two models of practice presented in the following chapter are generally referred to as ecological models because they conceptualize the person and environment as inseparable.

In some ways, both OPMA and PEOP could be seen as models that bridge the Chapters 3 and 4. Firstly, OPMA presents an understanding of the environment as intertwined with the person and mutually influencing, and therefore could have been placed with the ecological models. However, because of its structure borrowed from the occupational performance tradition, it was placed in this chapter to provide a comparison with OP. Similarly, PEOP conceptualizes the person and environment as more separate than the other two ecological models and presents occupation and performance as the mediums through which person and environment interact. However, unlike OA, it does not present the relationship between person and environment as one involving mastery. In Chapter 4, PEOP is placed first as it helps to provide a bridge between the models placed in this chapter and the ecological models included in the next.

## REFERENCES

American Occupational Therapy Association (AOTA), 2002. Occupational therapy practice framework: Domain and process. Am. J. Occup. Ther. 56, 609–639.

American Occupational Therapy Association (AOTA), 2008. Occupational therapy practice framework: Domain and process. Am. J. Occup. Ther. 62, 625–683.

Chapparo, C., Ranka, J., 1997. The Occupational Performance Model (Australia): A description of constructs and structure. In: Chapparo, C., Ranka, J. (Eds.), Occupational Performance Model (Australia): Monograph 1, Occupational Performance Network, Lidcombe, NSW.

Christiansen, C., Baum, C., 1997. Understanding occupation: definitions and concepts. In: Christiansen, C., Baum, C. (Eds.), Occupational therapy: Enabling function and well-being, second ed. Slack, Thorofare, NJ, pp. 3–25.

Department of National Health & Welfare (DNHW) & Canadian Association of Occupational Therapists (CAOT), 1983. Guidelines for the client-centred practice of occupational therapists. Cat. H39-33/1983E, Ottawa, ON.

Dunton, W., 1913. Occupation as a therapeutic measure. Med. Rec. 3, 388–389.

Gilfoyle, E., Grady, A., Moore, J., 1990. Children adapt. Slack, Thorofare, NJ.

Kielhofner, G., 1985. A model of human occupation: Theory and application. Williams & Wilkins, Baltimore, MD.

McHugh Pendleton, H., Schultz-Krohn, W., 2006. The occupational therapy practice framework and the practice of occupational therapy for people with physical disabilities. In: McHugh Pendleton, H., Schultz-Krohn, W. (Eds.), Occupational therapy: Practice skills for physical dysfunction, sixth ed. Mosby, St Louis, MI, pp. 2–16.

Meyer, A., 1922. The philosophy of occupational therapy. Arch. Occup. Ther. 1, 1–10.

Nelson, D., 1988. Occupation: Form and performance. Am. J. Occup. Ther. 42, 633–641.

Pedretti, L.W., 1996. Occupational Performance: A model for practice in physical dysfunction. In: Pedretti, L.W. (Ed.), Occupational therapy: Practice skills for physical dysfunction, fourth ed. Mosby, St Louis, MI, pp. 3–12.

Pedretti, L.W., Early, M.B. 2001. Occupational performance and models of practice for physical dysfunction. In: Pedretti, L.W., Early, M.B. (Eds.), Occupational therapy: Practice skills for physical dysfunction, fifth ed. Mosby, St Louis, MI, pp. 3–12.

Reed, K., 1984. Models of practice in occupational therapy. Williams & Wilkins, Baltimore, MD.

Schkade, J.K., McClung, M., 2001. Occupational Adaptation in practice: Concepts and cases. Slack, Thorofare, NJ.

Schkade, J.K., Schultz, S., 1992. Occupational Adaptation: Toward a holistic approach to contemporary practice, Part 1. Am. J. Occup. Ther. 46, 829–837.

Schkade, J.K., Schultz, S., 2003. Occupational Adaptation. In: Kramer, P., Hinosa, J., Royeen, C. (Eds.), Perspectives in human occupation. Lippincott Williams & Wilkins, Philadelphia, PA, pp. 181–221.

Schultz, S., 2009. Theory of Occupational Adaptation. In: Crepeau, E.B., Cohn, E.S., Boyt Schell, B.A. (Eds.), Willard & Spackman's occupational therapy, eleventh ed. Lippincott Williams & Wilkins, Philadelphia, PA, pp. 462–475.

Schultz, S., Schkade, J.K., 1992. Occupational Adaptation: Toward a holistic approach to contemporary practice, Part 2. Am. J. Occup. Ther. 46, 917–926.

Schultz, S., Schkade, J., 1997. Adaptation. In: Christiansen, C., Baum, C. (Eds.), Occupational therapy: Enabling function and well-being, second ed. Slack, Thorofare, NJ, pp. 459–481.

Occupational performance and adaptation models

Spencer, J., Davidson, H., 1998. Community adaptive planning assessment: A clinical tool for documenting future planning with clients. Am. J. Occup. Ther. 52, 19–30.

Spencer, J., Daybell, P.J., Eschenfelder, V., Khalaf, R., Pike, J.M., Woods-Pettitti, M., 1998. Contrasts in perspectives on work: An exploratory qualitative study based on the concept of adaptation. Am. J. Occup. Ther. 52, 474–484.

Spencer, J., Hersch, G., Eschenfelder, V., Fournet, J., Murray-Gerzik, M., 1999. Outcomes of protocol-based and adaptation-based occupational therapy interventions for low-income elderly persons on a transitional unit. Am. J. Occup. Ther. 53, 159–170.

White, V.K., 1998. Ethnic differences in the wellness of elderly persons. Occup. Ther. Health Care 11, 1–15.

# Person-environment-occupation models

4

## CHAPTER CONTENTS

As with most occupational therapy models, the models reviewed in this chapter centre on the influence of person, environment and occupation on people's abilities to act in the everyday world. However, these models emphasize the importance of the environment to a greater extent than the models reviewed in the previous chapter (with the proviso that the Occupational Performance Model (Australia) (OPMA) could have been placed in this chapter). Baum and Christiansen (2005) identified these types of models as person, environment, occupation or PEO models and Brown (2009) described them as ecological

© 2011 Elsevier Ltd.
DOI: 10.1016/B978-0-7234-3494-8.00004-8

models. They have also been described as transactional models as they emphasize the mutually influencing transaction that occurs between person and environment when engaged in occupation. The three models reviewed in this chapter are the Person-Environment-Occupation-Performance (PEOP) model by Christiansen and Baum, the Person-Environment-Occupation (PEO) model by Law and others, and the Ecology of Human Performance (EHP) by Dunn and others.

## PERSON-ENVIRONMENT-OCCUPATION-PERFORMANCE (PEOP) MODEL

We have placed this model first in the chapter as it appears to provide a bridge between the Occupational Performance (OP) model and ecological models. It acts as a bridge in sharing a trend with OP to analyze in detail the capacities of the individual. However, whereas OP provides comparatively little attention to the environment, the PEOP model provides a similar level of detail for analyzing the environment as it does for the person. The PEOP model was listed as an ecological model by Brown (2009). However, as discussed later in this chapter, this model differs from the other two models presented in this chapter through its conceptualization of the relationship between person, environment and occupation. In discussing this relationship, the other two models emphasize that person, environment and occupation should not be considered separately. The PEO emphasizes a transactive relationship between the three (rather than interactive) and EHP presents context as something through which person and occupation should be seen. Although similar to some of the other occupational therapy models, PEOP conceptualizes person and environment as joined by occupation (and performance and participation). That is, occupation is the medium through which person and occupation connect. In comparison with PEO, this model is interactive rather than transactive.

## MAIN CONCEPTS AND DEFINITIONS OF TERMS

The PEOP model is described as "a client-centred model organized to improve the everyday performance of necessary and valued occupations of individuals, organizations, and populations and their meaningful participation in the world around them" (Baum & Christiansen, 2005, p. 244). This definition demonstrates the importance of two concepts: occupational performance and participation in daily life. While many occupational therapy models explicitly focus on the enhancement of occupational performance as their main goal, this model explicitly identifies enhancing *participation* as a second primary goal. This model makes explicit that the goal of occupational performance is to enable participation in the social, cultural, financial and political world in which people and organizations exist. Therefore, a major contribution of the model is its acknowledgement that occupational performance might not be an end in itself but might gain meaning through its role in facilitating participation.

The focus of the model is the complex interaction between a person and his or her environment, which influences occupational performance and participation. This interaction forms the basis for occupation, in that intrinsic and extrinsic factors, respectively, form the foundation for what people

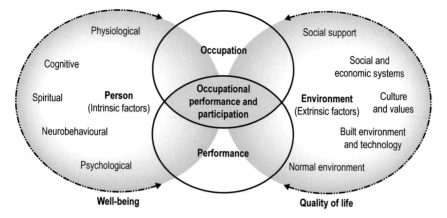

**FIG 4.1** Person-Environment-Occupation-Performance (PEOP) model. *Christiansen CH, Baum CM, Bass-Haugen J. Occupational Therapy: Performance, Participation and Well-Being, Third Edition, Thorofare, NJ: SLACK Incorporated; 2005. Reprinted with permission from SLACK Incorporated.*

do. Intrinsic factors (neurobehavioural, physiological, cognitive, psychological and emotional, and spiritual factors) and extrinsic factors (built, natural and cultural environments; societal factors; social interactions and social and economic systems) can "support, enable or restrict" (Baum & Christiansen, 2005, p. 244) performance by individuals, organizations and communities.

As suggested by its title, the four components of the model are person, environment, occupation and performance. Figure 4.1 shows the most recent diagram available at the time of publication. One useful way to think about this model is to interpret the four components (and diagram) as if lying in three dimensions. Upon a foundation of person and environment (first layer) lies occupation and performance (second layer) and on top of these are occupational performance and participation (third layer). First, *person* and *environment*, which interact in a mutually influencing way, form the foundation for what people do. The concept of 'person' includes the various capacities (neurobehavioural, psychological, etc.) that a person might have, which can influence what a person can and is inclined to do. These are referred to as *intrinsic factors*. The environment also has features that can affect performance (extrinsic factors). The *extrinsic factors* include physical, cultural and societal aspects of the context that surrounds them.

The second layer in the PEOP model comprises the components of occupational performance, that is, *occupation* and *performance*. The model makes clear distinctions between the concepts of occupation, performance and occupational performance, the last located in the third layer. Occupations were defined by Christiansen and Baum (2005) as "human pursuits that (a) are goal-directed or purposeful, (b) are performed in situations or contexts that influence how and with whom they are done, (c) can be identified by the doer and others, and (d) have individual meaning for the doer as well as shared meaning with others" (p. 5). They proposed that occupations can be classified according to what is done and how, why, where and when it is done. However, it is important to note here that occupation is not the same as performance. Where occupations and actions are done, performance refers to the actual doing of them. As Baum and Christiansen (2005) stated, "To be able to do requires that an action or a task be performed. Performance can come from either capacity intrinsic to the individual or by support provided by the environment or a combination of both." (p. 246.)

The top layer of the model, and the culmination of the previous layers, comprises *occupational performance* and *participation*. In the diagram provided, occupational performance and participation result where occupation and performance overlap. As Baum and Christiansen (2005) stated, "when occupation and performance are joined in the term occupational performance, it describes the actions that are meaningful to the individual as he or she cares for him- or herself, cares for others, works, plays, and participates fully in home and community life" (p. 246). In making the distinction between occupation, performance and occupational performance, they emphasized the meaning and purpose of occupational performance in the context of people's roles. Therefore, their statement that occupational performance is "the central construct of participation" (p. 246) places occupational performance within the context of meaningful and purposeful participation in an individual's broader societal context.

Baum and Christiansen's *hierarchy of occupation-related behaviours and supportive abilities* (2005; Christiansen & Baum, 1997a) is central to understanding the distinction between occupation and performance and occupational performance. This hierarchy places roles, occupations, tasks, actions and abilities in order from highest to lowest in complexity. As "occupations have a purpose" (Baum & Christiansen, 2005, p. 252), the top three levels on the hierarchy – roles, occupations and tasks – would be conceptualized in the *occupation* part of the model because they are linked to purpose. The next level in the hierarchy – actions – would be attended to in the *performance* part of the model, because they do not have a separate purpose. The lowest level of the hierarchy – abilities – would be considered in the *person* part of the model, as they lie within the person (as intrinsic factors). All of these occupation-related behaviours occur within a specific context or environment, which can support, enable or restrict the performance of occupations and tasks and, hence, affect participation in everyday life.

The model provides details of both person and environment, located in the first layer. A major technique in occupational therapy practice is the analysis of both person and environment for the purpose of facilitating occupational performance and participation. Therefore, this model provides substantial detail to guide occupational therapists in undertaking such analysis. The factors that contribute to a person's capacities are called intrinsic factors and those factors that relate to the context of occupational performance and participation are called extrinsic factors.

## INTRINSIC AND EXTRINSIC FACTORS

The intrinsic factors listed in the model (Baum & Christiansen, 2005) are physiological, cognitive, spiritual, neurobehavioural and psychological.

1. Physiological factors relate to a person's health and fitness. They include "abilities such as endurance, flexibility, movement, and strength" (p. 247) and are necessary for the performance of many tasks. Physiological factors contribute to and sustain health and well-being and can be enhanced by physical activity.
2. Cognitive factors are essential to "learning, communicating, moving, and observing" and include the "mechanisms of language comprehension and

production, pattern recognition, task organization, reasoning, attention, and memory" (p. 247). The authors claimed that occupational therapists need to understand the way experience affects the nervous system and how occupational performance can be used to facilitate cognitive rehabilitation. They stressed that attention to cognition should not be limited to situations where clients have cognitive impairment, but that occupational therapists should attend to the ways that particular occupations can maintain and promote these skills throughout the lifespan. They stated, "the link between cognition and occupation should be a central aspect of the interventions used to enhance and maintain health" (p. 247).

3. Spiritual factors refer to issues of meaning. Different objects and events have meaning for people. As Baum and Christiansen stated, "When these meanings contribute to a greater sense of personal understanding about self and one's place in the world, they can be described as spiritual" (p. 248). The creation of meaning requires a range of other intrinsic factors such as psychological and cognitive factors. Meanings are both shared and individual, in that, the shared meanings of the society influence the meanings that an individual attributes to an event or situation while meaning is also dependent on that individual's perspectives and experiences. The authors pointed out that everyday language is dependent upon the shared meanings of the culture but also influences thought.

4. Neurobehavioural factors refer to the sensory and motor systems that underlie performance. As Baum and Christiansen stated, "the ability to control movement, to modulate sensory input, to coordinate and integrate sensory information to compensate for sensorimotor deficits, and to modify neural structures through behaviour are all important characteristics that influence and support occupational performance [and participation]" (p. 248). By analyzing and using interventions based on neurobehavioural principles, occupational therapists can assist people to perform an occupation and participate in daily life.

5. Psychological factors are "the personality traits [interests, values, and attitudes that influence attention], motivational influences, and internal processes used by an individual to influence what they do, how these events are interpreted, and how they contribute to a sense of self" (p. 247). As this definition makes clear, psychological factors influence choice of occupation, interpretation of meaning and how a person thinks and feels about him- or herself. All of these processes affect occupational performance.

The external factors listed are social support, social and economic systems, culture and values, the built environment and technology, and the natural environment. The various external factors influence occupational performance and participation by placing demands or providing affordances.

1. Social support is experienced rather than observed and the amount of social support required varies from individual to individual. Three types of support have been identified. These are: practical support, informational support and emotional support. Practical support includes support that is tangible and is often referred to as instrumental support. Informational support includes the provision of advice, guidance and/or knowledge and skills training. Emotional support involves communicating regard and a sense of belonging and can involve the provision of emotional guidance.

2. Social and economic systems refer to the way the structure of society influences the resources available to particular individuals. The ways in which societies are structured advantage some groups and disadvantage other groups. People with disabilities are often disadvantaged in relation to social participation avenues such as employment. Baum and Christiansen made the point that "government and employment policies often dictate access to the resources that make doing possible" (p. 251) and discussed a range of organizations that have been established specifically to facilitate the social participation of people who are marginalized in some way. Baum and Christiansen suggested that "helping those individuals seek out resources to address their immediate needs, the occupational therapist can be an advocate for change in social and economic policies that create the societal limitations that impair the occupational performance of the total population" (p. 251).

3. Culture "refers to the values, beliefs, customs, and behaviours that are passed from one generation to the next. This includes socially transmitted behaviour patterns, arts, beliefs, institutions, and all other products of human work and thought" (p. 250). Culture shapes people's perspectives and attention and their attitudes towards and choice of occupation. Culture exists at all levels of society and can influence the attitudes, beliefs and behaviour of individuals, groups and populations. It can also affect structures such as organizations (organizational culture). Occupational therapists need to understand and attend to the influence of culture at all these levels and be sensitive to the beliefs and values of the people with whom they work.

4. The built environment and technology can facilitate or hinder occupational performance. It includes the various physical, sensory and design features of spaces that are built or developed by people (both private and public spaces). Technological features of the built environment include tools and appliances that support both action and rest. Examples include many of the basic appliances that are typical in households (e.g. television sets) as well as those referred to as assistive technology devices.

5. The natural environment includes "geographical features such as terrain, hours of sunlight, climate, and air quality" (p. 250). At times the natural environment creates necessary occupations (e.g. shovelling snow, walking to cover geographical distance to required resources) and the features of the natural environment can facilitate and hinder the ease with which various occupations are performed.

The internal and external environments are not inherently facilitatory or inhibitory. Occupational performance and participation are dependent upon the interaction between the internal and external factors in relation to the demands of the occupation being performed. This model provides substantial detail about both internal and external factors to support occupational therapists to analyze the interests, skills and capacities of the person, the demands of the environment and how they interact to facilitate or inhibit occupational performance and participation.

The PEOP is presented within the context of a larger text (as with CMOP-E, presented in the next chapter). The text, called *Occupational Therapy: Performance, Participation and Well-being* (Christiansen et al., 2005) relates to occupational therapy more generally and takes the reader through the fundamental assumptions of the profession relating to occupation before presenting the model. Thus, the PEOP forms one part of Christiansen's and Baum's broader conceptualization of occupation and occupational therapy.

This model commenced its development in 1985 (Baum & Christiansen, 2005). In 2005 the model was called Person-Environment-Occupation-Performance (PEOP) and it has undergone substantial changes and development in the three editions that were available at the time of publication. In each edition, it was called something different. The 1991 version was called a "Person-Environment-Performance" framework (Christiansen, 1991, p. 18) and was not referred to as a model. In 1997, it was called the "Person-Environment Occupational Performance Model" (Christiansen & Baum, 1997a). In 2005, it was called the "Person-Environment-Occupation-Performance Model" and provided with the acronym PEOP. The concepts of person, environment and performance appear to have remained the fundamental components of the model but the emphasis on occupation in the title as a separate concept has only recently emerged.

The distinction between occupation, performance and occupational performance is evident in all three editions of the model. The distinction between these concepts can be traced back to the model's use of Nelson's 1988 work, in which he distinguished between occupational form and performance. Christiansen (1991) stated, "all the elements comprising the context of the occupation are what Nelson (1988) terms *the form* of occupation. Occupational performance consists of *the doing* of occupation." (p. 27, italics in original.) In an adaptation of Nelson's work, Christiansen conceptualized occupational form as "the objective context of occupation consisting of: materials, environmental surround, other humans involved, temporal dimension, and sociocultural reality derived from social or cultural consensus" (p. 26).

In the first version, a binary distinction appears to have been made between the doing (performance) and a second concept (Christiansen's adaptation of occupational form) that includes what is done, the context in which it is done and the meaning of the doing to an individual. In this way, the first edition appears to have distinguished between performance and a broad conceptualization of occupational form, with the latter being ascribed meaning by an individual and occurring within a particular content.

In the second edition, a trio of concepts was presented. These were person, environment and occupational performance. This version emphasized that the performance of occupation is affected by a complex array of factors that influence performance, "as well as the many dimensions of occupation" (Christiansen & Baum, 1997a, p. 49). Christiansen and Baum stated, "Occupational performance consists of the 'doing' of occupation; whereas occupational form concerns the context of the doing" (1997b, p. 6).

In the second edition, the concept of occupational form has been explicitly presented as involving the interaction between person and environment. This is consistent with Christiansen's earlier interpretation of Nelson's concept of occupational form to include the meaning that the occupation has for an individual. In the second edition, the concept of occupation is like the invisible focus of the model. Using the metaphor of the window presented in the Introduction, occupation is like the window through which one might look without making the window itself explicit in the description of what one sees. Consequently, the concept of occupation was not specifically included in the diagrammatic representations of the model but was integral to it, in that it was present in all three parts of the model – person, environment and occupational performance.

In the first and second editions, the concept of occupational form appears to have been separated into person and environment (conceptualized as mutually influencing) and contrasted with performance. By the third edition of the model, the separation of concepts is most obvious. In that version, the capacities of an individual and the context in which something is done (sociocultural and physical environment) are presented as separate but mutually influencing. They provide the background to the occupation and its performance, which combine to result in occupational performance and participation.

In the second edition, the model emphasized the importance of occupational performance to self-identity and a sense of fulfilment. (However, this emphasis might have become lost in the most recent edition or at least become subsumed under the concept of participation.) In the second edition, Christiansen and Baum (1997a) stated, "over time, these meaningful experiences permit people to develop an understanding of who they are and what their place is in the world" (p. 48).

This focus on self-identity, combined with the detailed explication of personal factors such as motivation, values and meaning, emphasizes the biopsychosocial nature of occupational therapy practice, as conveyed in this edition of the model. This focus is consistent with the link that is made between occupational performance (highlighted as function rather than impairment) and well-being (rather than just health), which are also consistent with a biopsychosocial approach to health. The second edition also provided a table showing the relationship between the "intrinsic performance enablers" that the model conceptualized as factors intrinsic to the person and the well-accepted occupational therapy concept of "performance components". These intrinsic factors remained present in the third edition of the model and distinguish it from other PEO models such as the model published by Law et al., described later in this chapter.

In all three versions of the PEOP model (with various different names), the model is linked to both a hierarchy of occupational performance and the WHO classification of the time. In the 1991 version, this hierarchy is presented (from lowest to highest) as activities, tasks and roles. In the second and third editions (1997 & 2005), the hierarchy presents abilities, actions, tasks, occupations and roles. The first and second editions of the model are linked to the International Classification of Impairments, Disabilities and Handicaps (ICIDH) and the third edition to the International Classification of Functioning, Disability and Health (ICF).

The PEOP is the third edition of the model of practice created by Charles Christiansen and Carolyn Baum. The model conceptualizes the focus of occupational therapy as occupational performance and participation. It provides guidance for practice by breaking down these concepts into the components of occupation and performance and by identifying the factors internal to the person and within the environment that influence occupational performance and participation. All four components of the model are seen as separate but interacting. The PEOP model has similarities with the OP model through the way it breaks down factors internal to the person. However, its focus on the environment and the external factors that influence occupational performance and participation are more extensive than in the OP model. Therefore, it has been described as a person, environment, occupation model.

4

Person-environment-occupation models

See Box 4.1.

---

**BOX 4.1 Person-Environment-Occupation-Performance (PEOP) model memory aid**

- What do these people want or need to do in their daily lives (occupation) and can these tasks, occupations and roles be done (performance) successfully by these people in the current context (occupational performance and participation)?

- What roles (social responsibilities & privileges) do these people have and want to or intend to continue with?

- What occupations have meaning for these people and how would it affect their roles if they were unable to perform them?

**Intrinsic factors**
What factors (performance enablers) intrinsic to these people (person) affect their capability to perform specific occupations in context?

**Extrinsic factors**
What factors extrinsic to these people (environment) affect their capacity to perform specific occupations in context?

How do these factors support, enable or restrict the performance of roles, occupations, tasks & actions?

**Checklist**
Neurobehavioural factors
- Sensory (olfactory, gustatory, visual, auditory, somatosensory, proprioceptive, vestibular)
- Motor (somatic, cerebellum, basal ganglia network, thalamic integration)

Physiological factors
- Endurance, flexibility, movement, strength

**Checklist**
The built environment
- Physical properties (accessibility, manageability, safety, aesthetics)
- Tools & appliances

The natural environment
- Geographical features (terrain, sunlight, climate, air quality)

---

## Intrinsic factors

Cognitive factors

■ Language comprehension &
production, pattern recognition,
task organization, reasoning,
attention, memory

Psychological and emotional factors

■ Self-identity (self-concept,
self-esteem, self-efficacy), sense
of well-being, interests, values &
attitudes that influence attention,
behaviour & interpretation of
events

Spiritual factors

■ Individual and shared meanings

## Extrinsic factors

The cultural environment

■ Expected norms for time & space
use, behaviour, activity
■ Social role expectations
(age, gender)
■ Shared explanations for health and
well-being and ill health.

Societal factors

■ Social acceptance, stereotyping &
attitudes to difference, stigma
(social prejudice)

Social interaction

■ Practical support (instrumental, aid,
tangible support), informational
support (advice, guidance,
knowledge, skill training), and
emotional support (communicates
esteem & belonging, provides
guidance)

Social and economic systems

■ Economic security and/or
independence
■ Availability of and access to
resources (housing, employment,
technology
■ Infrastructure, policies and
legislation affecting participation

Person-environment-occupation models

Baum, C., Christiansen, C., 2005. Person-Environment-Occupation-Performance: An occupation-based framework for practice. In: Christiansen, C.H., Baum, C.M., Bass-Haugen, J. (Eds.), Occupational therapy: Performance, participation, and well-being, third ed. Slack, Thorofare, NJ, pp. 243–259.

Christiansen, C., 1991. Occupational therapy: Intervention for life performance. In: Christiansen, C., Baum, C. (Eds.), Occupational therapy: Overcoming human performance deficits. Slack, Thorofare, NJ, pp. 3–43.

Christiansen, C., Baum, C., 1997a. Person-Environment-Occupational Performance: A conceptual model for practice. In: Christiansen, C., Baum, C. (Eds.), Occupational therapy: Enabling function and well-being, second ed. Slack, Thorofare, NJ, pp. 47–70.

Christiansen, C., Baum, C., 1997b. Understanding occupation: Definitions and concepts. In: Christiansen, C., Baum, C. (Eds.), Occupational therapy: Enabling function and well-being, second ed. Slack, Thorofare, NJ, pp. 3–25.

## PERSON-ENVIRONMENT-OCCUPATION MODEL OF OCCUPATIONAL PERFORMANCE

The next two models presented in this chapter are informed by the concepts relating to human ecology. Both models were published in the mid-1990s, within 2 years of each other. The first model of practice presented is the Person-Environment-Occupation (PEO) model (Law et al., 1996). As the name suggests, the major concepts in this model of practice are person, environment and occupation, which provide a way of understanding occupational performance when considered together. The concept of person-environment-occupation fit is used to outline the relationship between these different elements. When the three 'fit' together well, it enhances occupational performance. However, when there is a poor alignment between the three, occupational performance is reduced.

## MAIN CONCEPTS AND DEFINITIONS OF TERMS

This model of practice was based on the literature on human ecology at the time of its publication. Human ecology is concerned with the relationship between human beings and their environment. As is evident in the models reviewed in this book, attention to the relationship between person and environment was a consistent feature in publications about occupational therapy models during the 1990s (both those developed during this time and the 1990s versions of those with multiple editions). This 1990s emphasis on understanding the person in the context of their environments probably represents the crystallizations of ideas that had been percolating during the 1970s and 1980s. It constitutes a move away from a biomedical model of health to a biopsychosocial model, where individuals are seen within their broader context (the broader systems that surround them).

PEO conceptualizes the relationship between the person and the environment as "transactive" (Law et al., 1996, p. 10) rather than interactive (as with PEOP). The distinction between these two concepts relates to whether person and environment are conceptualized as distinct entities that could be studied separately or whether they should be examined together. An interactive approach would take the former position and consider the two as separate entities that are able to be measured separately and that influence the other in a cause and effect way. As Law et al. explained, "An interactive approach allows behaviour to be predicted and controlled, by influencing change at the level of an individual or environmental characteristic" (p. 10). In contrast, a transactive approach presents the person and environment as interdependent and proposes that a person's behaviour cannot be separated from the context within which it occurs (including temporal, physical and psychological factors). Therefore, occupational performance is a context-, person- and occupation-specific process. That is, it is the result of particular people doing particular things in particular times and places.

The relationship between person and environment is understood to be mutually influencing. As Law et al. (1996) stated, "a person's contexts are continually shifting and as contexts change, the behaviour necessary to accomplish a goal also changes" (p. 10). Therefore, rather than person and environment being examined separately, in a transactive approach, an *event* becomes the unit of study. As such, the observable features of the environment in which the event took place would be investigated as well as the event's meaning to those participating. This process provides for a rich understanding of the interconnectedness of person and environment and helps to provide an understanding of how a person's behaviour shapes and is shaped by the environment.

It is important within this model to understand the distinction made between interactive and transactive approaches to the person–environment relationship because the diagram of three overlapping circles (person, environment and occupation), which has probably become most associated with this model, could be misconstrued as representing an interactive rather than transactive approach (because it presents person, environment and occupation as separate but overlapping entities). However, in its published form, a three-dimensional atom-like diagram was presented, which makes the interconnectedness of these three elements clear (Figure 4.2). The diagram shows three interconnected components – environmental supports and barriers, individual skills, and occupational demands – surrounding occupational performance. Occupational performance is considered to be the "outcome of the transaction of the person, environment and occupation. It is defined as the dynamic experience of a person engaged in purposeful activities and tasks within an environment." (Law et al., 1996, p. 16.)

The first component of the model that we will discuss is *person*. The biopsychosocial understanding of the person is evident in discussions where Law et al. (1996) explain that occupational performance can be measured both objectively and subjectively. That is, there are features that can be observed and recorded in an objective way as well as features that relate to the experiences of the performer. The authors advocated that the latter be measured through methods such as self-report.

The changing nature of subjective experience and views of self is central to the concept of the person in this model. The person is presented as "a dynamic, motivated and ever-developing being, constantly interacting with the environment" (p. 17). People change over time as the environments surrounding

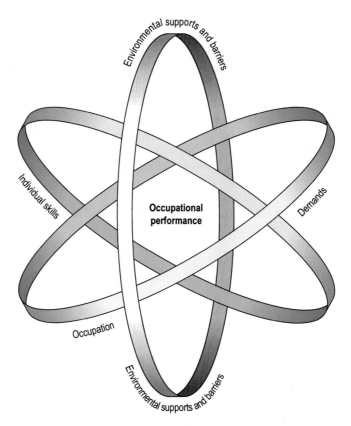

**FIG 4.2** Person-Environment-Occupation atom diagram. *From Law M., Cooper B., Strong S., Stewart D., Rigby P., Letts L., The person-environment-occupation model: A transactive approach to occupational performance, 1996, Canadian Journal of Occupational Therapy, 63(1), 9–23. Reprinted with the permission of CAOT Publications ACE.*

them change. They change in their attributes, characteristics, abilities and skills and in the ways they think and feel about themselves. Their sense of who they are and what they are capable of develops and changes as they interact with the specific environments that surround them.

Consistent with the richly connected and contextualized view of the person is a broad definition of *environment*. As Law et al. (1996) stated, "the broad definition gives equal importance to the considerations of the environment" (p. 16). While occupational therapists have traditionally emphasized the influence of the physical environment on what people do and how they do it, this model makes explicit that a range of environmental considerations are equally important in influencing human behaviour and activity. While this broad concept of the environment is consistent with other models published in the 1990s, its uniqueness lies in its emphasis on the transactive relationship between the environment and person. The only other model that emphasized this degree of interconnectedness was the Ecology of Human Performance (Dunn et al., 1994).

The model outlines five aspects of the context surrounding the person – cultural, socioeconomic, institutional, physical and social – that shape and are shaped by that person. For example, culture shapes what people believe and how they see the world. This, in turn, shapes how they think about themselves and what they might want and/or are expected to do. However, individuals' views of the world and of themselves are also dependent upon the degree to which each individual internalizes the views of the culture and the people surrounding them. What they actually do, then, influences and is influenced by the environment within which they act. Their socioeconomic circumstances will also influence their perception of what they can and can't do as well as their access to resources. Just as a person grows and ages and changes in their skills, abilities, character and experiences, so too their circumstances are likely to change over the course of their lives. Environments can change because people physically relocate; change their roles, habits and routines; change their social and cultural groupings, etc. or because local, national and world circumstances change. For example, the environment surrounding a person living at the beginning of the twentieth century will differ greatly from that of a person living during the twenty-first century.

The third aspect of the model considers what people do within their environmental contexts. While this is called *occupation* in the model's name, Law et al. (1996) considered three aspects of human action – activity, task and occupation – under this category. They presented these three concepts as "nested within each other" (p. 16) and claimed that they drew upon the work of Christiansen and Baum (1991) in their categorization (note: Christiansen's and Baum's most recent hierarchy does not use the word activity at all, possibly because there is a lack of consensus about whether activity is a component of a task or vice versa). Activity was defined as "a singular pursuit in which a person engages as part of his/her daily occupational experience" and was considered to be "the basic unit of a task" (p. 16). They gave the example of the act of handwriting. Task was defined as "a set of purposeful activities in which a person engages" and could be represented by "the obligation to write a report" (p. 16). Occupation, then, was considered as "groups of self-directed, functional tasks and activities in which a person engages over the lifespan" (p. 16). To continue with the same example, Law et al. suggested that occupation would be "a managerial position requiring an individual to engage in frequent report writing" (p. 16), which might constitute one of their professional activities.

Law et al. (1996) further defined "occupations" (the plural) as "those clusters of activities and tasks in which the person engages in order to meet his/her intrinsic needs for self-maintenance, expression and fulfilment" (p. 16) and explained that they are linked to roles and conducted in the context of multiple environments. This definition emphasizes that self-maintenance, expression and fulfilment are understood as intrinsic needs and that people engage in occupations within the context of their specific roles and environments. It is these roles and environments that shape the process and purpose of occupations for a particular person.

*Occupational performance* results from the interconnectedness of the person, what he/she is aiming to do and where it will be done. However, the rich connections between these three factors are evident when realizing that even individuals' decisions about what to do are shaped by the broader context in which they live their lives. Occupational performance is the result of a complex process in which people determine the purpose of occupations in their

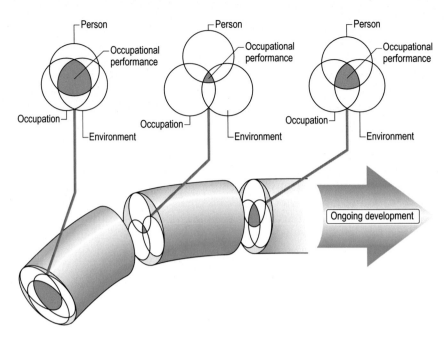

FIG 4.3   **Person-Environment-Occupation lifespan diagram.** *From Law M., Cooper B., Strong S., Stewart D., Rigby P., Letts L., The person-environment-occupation model: A transactive approach to occupational performance, 1996, Canadian Journal of Occupational Therapy, 63(1), 9–23. Reprinted with the permission of CAOT Publications ACE.*

lives; a process that is shaped by their perceptions, goals, responsibilities and desires and the demands of the context in which they live. In a reciprocal way, how they think about themselves and the things people do also influence their environments. Occupational performance also changes over time, as represented in Figure 4.3, as the relationship between person, environment and occupation changes through the lifespan and will differ at different times for any particular person.

Central to the model is the concept of the person-environment-occupation fit. The degree of congruence between these three elements affects occupational performance. As Law et al. (1996) stated, "the outcome of greater compatibility is therefore represented as more optimal occupational performance" (p. 17). When the congruence between them diminishes, occupational performance is impeded. In Figure 4.3, three circles overlapped to different extents represents this process. As evident in the diagram, these overlapping circles come from a cross-section of the diagram used to represent the temporal aspects of occupational performance throughout the lifespan. The effect of greater or lesser congruence between person, environment and occupation on occupational performance is apparent. The goal of occupational therapy is to improve occupational performance (if it is reduced) by facilitating or enhancing the fit between person, environment and occupation.

Written at a time when a systems approach and the biopsychosocial model of health were prominent ideas, the PEO particularly emphasized that occupational performance was person-, environment- and occupation-specific and that the three could not be considered separately. Consequently, intervention

4

USING OCCUPATIONAL THERAPY MODELS IN PRACTICE

104

could be targeted at any one or more of the three elements, as a change in one would be expected to lead to a change in the others. However, it is important to note that a transactive understanding of the relationship among the three components means that, while a change is expected, the exact nature of that change *cannot be predicted*.

At the time, Law et al. (1996) listed four advantages of using the PEO Model of Occupational Performance. These were that:

1. it enables people to select from and use interventions that are directed at person, occupation and environment in different ways;
2. it provides a framework for using multiple paths (in conjunction) to effect change;
3. it draws particular attention to interventions that address different levels of the environment and the importance of selecting and implementing interventions "in context"; and
4. by taking an ecological approach to the environment, it provides for the "use of a wider repertoire of well validated instruments of measure developed by other disciplines" (p. 18).

## HISTORICAL DESCRIPTION OF MODEL'S DEVELOPMENT

There is a certain level of symmetry in placing a transactional model, which assumes that action takes place within a particular context, within its particular historical and geographical context. This model was published in 1996, a decade in which occupational therapy models were commonly emphasizing occupational therapy's assumption that people should be understood in a holistic way. That is, they should be understood as both 'whole' people (rather than just bodies) and people who live in a particular context (their 'whole' situation). Placed within the broader context of models of health, it was a time when a biopsychosocial understanding of health was becoming more established, in contrast to the biomedical understanding characteristic of the preceding period.

Law et al. (1996) claimed that the importance of the relationship between person and environment had been well recognized during the profession's early history but not emphasized from the 1940s to the 1960s (a time Reed, 2005, described as the mechanistic period and characterized by the 'forgetting' of many formative concepts). Law et al. summed up this view of the situation by saying, "Occupational performance results from the dynamic relationship between people, their occupations and roles, and the environments in which they live, work and play. There have, however, been few models of practice in the occupational therapy literature which discuss the theoretical and clinical applications of person-environment interaction" (p. 9). Presumably, the authors saw the need for occupational therapy to make explicit its contextualized understanding of human occupation.

The main publication presenting this model appeared in the *Canadian Journal of Occupational Therapy* in 1996. In providing their rationale for the model, Law et al. (1996) argued that occupational therapy's "views on the relationship between occupation and the environment have altered" (p. 10), in that they had moved away from the cause and effect assumptions inherent within a biomedical model of health and moved towards a more "transactive" (p. 10) understanding of occupational performance. They also provided a literature review, highlighting key publications that demonstrated "the importance of the environment in influencing behaviour and the use of the environment as a treatment modality in occupational therapy" (p. 13). They noted that this concern had been increasingly discussed from the mid-1980s to the mid-1990s. Thus, they placed the model within the existing trends in occupational therapy.

This placing of the model within existing trends might suggest that the authors were aiming to describe the theory and practice of occupational therapy at the time, rather than intending to shape it into a new understanding. (This is different from some of the other models reviewed in this book, which do appear to have the aim of shaping occupational therapy theory and practice in particular ways.) If this assumption is correct, it might help to explain why this model is so well known and used, despite having only been published in one major article. That is, it may have provided occupational therapists with a language and concepts for describing what they believed about their theory and practice related to occupation. Certainly, the concepts of person, environment and occupation being interdependent and mutually influencing have become central to occupational therapy discourse about human action in the intervening years.

Law et al. (1996) also explained that "the previous medical orientation of practice has linked occupational therapy more naturally with other health professionals and not necessarily fostered interaction with social scientists, human geographers, architects and interior designers, interested in planning therapeutic and enabling environments" (p. 14). This is an interesting statement to reflect upon more than two decades later, when we have seen similar sentiments expressed by those advocating for an occupational science approach and we also see the healthcare context having changed to incorporate a broader view of health and the proliferation of occupational therapists working in areas other than health.

## SUMMARY

The PEO model presents the three major components of occupational therapy's domain of concern (person, environment and occupation) and conceptualizes their relationship as transactive. This means that they should not be considered separately but are considered mutually influencing, in that a change in any one or more domains leads to a change in the others. While such change is expected, the model suggests that the exact nature of the change cannot be predicted or controlled (a change will definitely occur but a particular type of change cannot be predetermined). The degree to which these three components *fit* together influences occupational performance. That is, if the congruence among person-environment-occupation is high, then occupational performance will be enhanced. If the fit is poor, occupational performance is reduced. The aim of occupational therapy is to facilitate occupational performance by intervening in any one or more of these areas to enhance the congruence between person, environment and occupation.

See Box 4.2.

---

**BOX 4.2  Person-Environment-Occupation Model of Occupational Performance (PEO) memory aid**

What *events* are relevant to this client? (What does this *person* need/want to *do* in the *context* of his/her life?)

■ What occupation is required?

■ Who will do it?

■ What does it mean to that person?

■ In what environment and under what circumstances will it be done?

How is/has the cultural, socioeconomic, institutional, physical and social environment shaping/shaped that perception?

How is he/she performing those activities, tasks and occupations (objective measures)?

How does he/she experience performing those activities, tasks and occupations (subjective measures)?

What degree of congruence exists between:

■ the person's abilities, perceptions and experiences;

■ the cultural, socioeconomic, institutional, physical and social environment; and

■ the activities, tasks and occupations that are being/need to be performed?

What combination of interventions might assist in increasing the congruence between person, environment and occupation?

Where should those interventions be targeted (person, environment, occupation)?

---

Law, M., Cooper, B., Strong, S., 1996. The Person-Environment-Occupation Model: A transactive approach to occupational performance. Can. J. Occup. Ther. 63 (1), 9–23.

## ECOLOGY OF HUMAN PERFORMANCE

Ecology of Human Performance (EHP) is the second model that conceptualizes the environment as an inseparable aspect of occupation. That is, it is the context within which people act and which shapes and is shaped by that action. As the name suggests, the model is informed by the principles of ecology. It was developed at a similar time to the PEO and published 2 years earlier.

## MAIN CONCEPTS AND DEFINITIONS OF TERMS

EHP emphasizes the environment as the primary context within which performance needs to be understood. It is a lens through which all human performance should be viewed. The term ecology refers to the "interrelationships of organisms and their environments" (Dunn et al., 1994, p. 595) and the model emphasizes the inter relatedness of person, context, task and performance. The model was first published in 1994. In the original publication, the authors stated, "the primary theoretical postulate fundamental to the EHP framework is that ecology, or the interaction between person and the environment, affects human behaviour and performance, and that performance cannot be understood outside of context" (p. 598). Thus, context is central to human performance. Figure 4.4 provides a diagrammatic representation of EHP. In this model (Dunn, 2007) there are three important constructs – person, task and context (initially called environment) – which contribute to an understanding of the fourth construct: human performance.

A central feature of this model is the primary importance to human performance of *environment* or *context*. The model conceptualizes the environment as the broader context that is integral to and shapes both the person and his or her task performance (not limited to the physical context in which a task is performed). This understanding of the environment has two aspects that need to be considered in more depth. These are: (a) that the environment includes more than just the physical environment; and (b) that the environment has the capacity to shape task performance.

First, while the earlier publications of the model use the term environment (or context-environment), the authors articulated very clearly that the term is conceptualized very broadly and should not be limited to the physical environment. They stated that the concept of the environment should be expanded to include, "physical, temporal, social, and cultural elements" (Dunn et al., 1994, p. 596). By expanding the definition of environment in this way, Dunn et al. emphasized the contribution that occupational therapists can make to an understanding of the interdependent relationship between

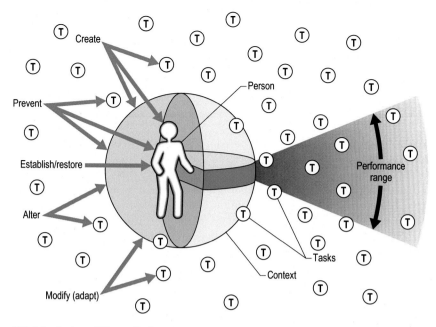

FIG 4.4  **Ecology of Human Performance.** *Reprinted from Dunn in Kramer (1994),* Perspectives in Human Occupation, *with permission from Lippincott, Williams and Wilkins.*

the person and environment. They claimed that a broad definition of environment helps to make explicit the complexity of the person–environment relationship to a level that is beyond the scope of the work done by environmental psychologists (who mainly focused on the physical environment). In particular, a broader concept of the environment allows occupational therapists to consider the meaning of the physical, temporal, social and cultural environment to the person.

Second, while the influence of the environment on human performance has long been acknowledged in occupational therapy, the EHP model emphasizes that the environment also shapes both the person and the tasks in which the person engages. In a review of the social science literature on the effect of the environment, Dunn et al. (1994, p. 596) cited a range of different authors and the main emphasis of their work. These included:

- Jerome Bruner (1989), who conceptualized the environment as providing a context for the construction of the self;
- Lawton (1982), who applied Murray's (1938) concept of environmental press, emphasizing that the demands of the environment influence a person's perceptions of his or her own competence; and
- Gibson's (1986) phenomenological approach to perception, whereby people's perceptions of objects in the environment are influenced by the opportunities that the environment affords them.

These are just a few of the ideas that influenced the EHP's concept of the importance of the environment in shaping how people view themselves and what they do.

As the focus of the model is the relationship between person and environment, the second construct that we will discuss here is *person*. Dunn et al (2003) stated that "the Ecology of Human Performance is an individually focused, client-centred framework. Individuals are seen as unique and complex" (p. 225). Personal variables contribute to the uniqueness of individuals. These are listed in the model as values, interests and experiences, as well as sensorimotor, cognitive and psychosocial skills. These personal variables influence both the selection of tasks and the quality of task performance. These personal variables are also continually influenced by the person's (continually changing) context.

The third construct is *task*. The model takes the view that a multitude of tasks are potentially available to all people. These are represented in Figure 4.4 by the capital Ts that lie outside of the person-context sphere. However, personal and environmental variables influence the tasks that form part of an individual's actual repertoire of tasks. Personal variables such as interests, values, perceptions and experience as well as sensorimotor, cognitive and psychosocial skills and abilities influence the selection of tasks in which the person participates. Environmental variables also influence task selection and performance. For example, some tasks might not be easily accessed in certain environments such as snow skiing in a temperate climate while others might not be socially or culturally valued. In addition, a person might engage in a selection of tasks because the context 'requires' these tasks of them. Examples include those tasks that are required in order to fulfil the particular social roles expected of the person. The set of tasks in which a particular person engages will depend on the unique relationship between the person and his or her specific context. This set of tasks is referred to as the *performance range* and people select from the available range of tasks. The performance range is influenced by a person's skills and abilities and the supports and barriers created by the particular context. As people and contexts change, so too do their performance ranges.

The final construct in the model is *human performance*. This is the result of the interaction between person, context and task.

## INTERVENTIONS

In addition to the four core constructs already discussed, EHP also addresses five categories of interventions. These are establish/restore, alter, adapt, prevent and create. These five alternatives for intervention relate variously to person, context and task.

First, therapeutic interventions can aim to *establish* or *restore* an individual's skills and abilities. This intervention refers to either establishing skills that people haven't had previously or restoring skills and abilities that have been lost, usually through acquiring a medical condition, injury or disability. Dunn et al. (1994) made the point that restorative interventions are very common among occupational therapists working within a biomedical model, with its corrective emphasis. While these interventions target the individual's skills and abilities, Dunn et al. stressed that context can be important in these types of intervention and gave the example of the importance of predictable environments in the provision of feedback for correcting motor behaviours.

The second way that occupational therapists might intervene is to *alter* or *change* the actual environment, that is, to select a different environment in which the person is able to perform the task. This intervention aims to create the best match between the person and his or her environment and focuses on selecting a different environment rather than adapting the current environment (i.e. not to be confused with altering or making changes to the current environment).

The third intervention alternative is to *adapt* the contextual features and/or task demands. Regarding contextual features, these could be enhanced or minimized to match better the person's abilities. Similarly, aspects of the task such as the sequence of steps, the tools used, the position required of the person and the skills required of the person can be adapted to enable the person to participate in the task.

The fourth intervention alternative is to *prevent*. In this option, occupational therapists might aim to "prevent the occurrence or evolution of maladaptive performance in context" (Dunn et al., 1994, p. 604). This intervention strategy aims to prevent difficulties arising. To do this, occupational therapists might address person, context and/or task.

The final intervention option is called *create* and was described by Dunn et al. as "creating circumstances that promote more adaptable or complex performance in context" (p. 604). The authors stressed that this intervention does not assume the presence of a disability or that there is a problem that will interfere with performance.

## HISTORICAL DESCRIPTION OF MODEL'S DEVELOPMENT

Like PEO, EHP was developed at a time when the profession was making more explicit its fundamental assumptions about the importance of the environment in occupational performance. In many ways, the 1990s could be seen as a time in occupational therapy's history where the reductionism of the mechanistic period was increasingly being critiqued and many of occupational therapy's fundamental beliefs were being reaffirmed.

The EHP model was developed by the Department of Occupational Therapy at the University of Kansas, originally for three reasons outlined by Dunn (2007). These were:

1. to produce a framework that would support and guide the scholarly work produced by that department;
2. to provide a means for organizing their curriculum and communicating their perspectives to their students; and
3. (most importantly, according to Dunn) to develop a framework to support the planning of work conducted in conjunction with their interdisciplinary colleagues.

According to Dunn, the EHP model was successful in supporting all three original aims. At the time that the model was developed, the authors (Dunn et al., 1994) explained that, while the environment had been "a recurring theme in the occupational therapy literature" (p. 595), insufficient attention had been made to the influence of contextual features on human performance. Dunn (2007) also emphasized that, at the time, the context had also been neglected by other services as well as occupational therapy.

In the three major publications on this model between 1994 and 2007, the model has undergone very little change. The major difference is really one of categorization, in that, the original version of the model included "therapeutic intervention" as a fifth construct in the practice of occupational therapy (in addition to person, task, context and occupational performance). While intervention was not listed as a separate construct in later versions of the model, the five different intervention strategies outlined in the earlier version (establish/restore, alter, adapt, prevent and create) have remained an integral part of the model.

In discussing the development of the model, Dunn (2007) emphasized the conscious decision not to use the term "occupation" in the EHP model. This was because one of its original purposes was to provide a framework from which to work with colleagues outside the discipline of occupational therapy and the authors thought the particular way that occupational therapists use the term occupation could make this process difficult. Instead, the term "task" was used, as the developers were of the opinion it had utility and a common understanding within everyday language. However, in the later publications, the concept of occupation, which had very much taken root in occupational therapy discourse by then, was discussed more overtly. For example, in explaining the choice to use the word task in a 2007 publication, Dunn emphasized that the "construct of occupation" (p. 128), whereby a person derives meaning from performance of a task in context, is important to understanding human performance.

While EHP has gone through little change or development over time, it has had a broad influence on occupational therapy. In 2007, Dunn stated, "One of the most helpful benefits of including context is that intervention options expand" (p. 128). Interestingly, the five intervention approaches that they identified in 1994 – establish/restore, adapt/modify, alter, prevent and create – appear to have influenced the American Occupational Therapy Association's Occupational Therapy Practice Framework (AOTA, 2002, 2008), as these five appear unchanged in that document as treatment planning and implementation strategies.

## SUMMARY

EHP is an ecological model of occupational therapy that emphasizes the context through which task performance should be viewed. Whereas other models of practice in occupational therapy generally start with the person and focus on occupational performance in context, this model starts with context. Using the image of the window presented in the Introduction, it is as if *context* is the window through which the model looks at occupational performance. In contrast, the window in most other occupational therapy models is generally occupation, with the variation between models relating to whether they include the window in the description of what is seen or not.

The model was first published in 1994 and has changed very little in the three major publications in which it has been presented. The primary focus of the model is the person in context. This person in context has a range of tasks available to them and this range is influenced by both person and context. The role of occupational therapy is to identify this performance range of available tasks and determine whether it meets the needs of the person in that context. The model outlines five intervention options:

1. to *establish* or *restore* an individual's skills and abilities;
2. to *alter* the actual environment, that is, to select a different environment in which the person is able to perform the task;
3. to *adapt* the contextual features and/or task demands;
4. to *prevent* the development or maintenance of problems in occupational performance in context; and
5. to *create* circumstances that promote valued occupational performance in context.

See Box 4.3.

---

**BOX 4.3  Ecology of Human Performance memory aid**

**In this situation:**
Who is the relevant person?

- What are their experiences; interests; sensorimotor, cognitive & psychosocial skills (and how have these changed or are likely to change)?

- In what ways does the context shape him/her or he/she shape the context?

- How do his/her abilities/skills/interests affect task selection and performance

What are the relevant contexts?

- temporal environment (e.g. age, life cycle, time in history)?

- physical environment?

- social environment?

- cultural environment?

- how well do these match the person's abilities/interests/skills and the tasks that need to be done?

- how are these contexts likely to change?

What are the relevant tasks (sets of behaviour, could be components of occupation)?

- what tasks are available to the person?

- how well do the tasks match the person's abilities/skills/interests?

- what tasks are available in the relevant contexts?

**Intervention planning**
Which intervention methods could be used to facilitate successful participation and where will they be aimed?

| | |
|---|---|
| ■ Establish/restore | Personal skills & abilities |
| ■ Alter (different environment) | Context (environmental variables) |
| ■ Adapt/modify | Context (environmental variables) |
| | Task (demands of) |
| | Context (environmental variables) |
| ■ Prevent (anticipate problem) | Personal variables |
| | Task variables |
| | Context (environmental variables) |
| ■ Create | Personal variables |
| | Task variables |
| | Context (environmental variables) |

## MAJOR WORKS

Dunn, W., 2007. Ecology of Human
Performance Model. In: Dunbar, S.B.
(Ed.), Occupational therapy models for
intervention with children and families.
Slack, Thorofare, NJ, pp. 127–155.
Dunn, W., Brown, C., McQuigan, A., 1994.
The ecology of human performance:
A framework for considering the effect
of context. Am. J. Occup. Ther. 48 (7),
595–607.
Dunn, W., Brown, C., Youngstrom, M.J.,
2003. Ecological model of occupation.
In: Kramer, P., Hinojosa, J., Royeen, C.B.
(Eds.), Perspectives in human occupation:
participation in life. Lippincott Williams &
Wilkins, Baltimore, MD, pp. 222–263.

## CONCLUSION

In this chapter we reviewed three models of practice that are often referred to as ecological because of the particular emphasis they place on the environment. The PEOP model was presented first as it could be considered to provide a bridge between the occupational performance models and the more deeply ecological models. The PEOP is unique in that it provides substantial detail about the capacities of the individual that affect performance while also providing substantial detail about the environmental context. Both person and environment are presented as two equally important and mutually influencing factors upon which people perform occupation for the purpose of occupational performance and participation in society.

The PEO model has become widely known and there has been broad acceptance of the importance of person, environment and occupation in occupational therapy theory and practice more generally. The idea that person, environment and occupation are tied together in a transactive relationship is central to the model, the implication being that they cannot be considered separately. Ecology of Human Performance also presents the environment as something *through which* occupational performance must be understood.

These ecological approaches to occupational therapy have been important influences in shaping the profession's understanding of occupation. The importance of the environment as central to occupation and its performance has become well accepted in the broader occupational therapy discourse. In Chapter 5, the CMOP-E is presented. This model introduces another important concept that may shape occupational therapy thinking in the future. That is the importance of a just society.

## REFERENCES

American Occupational Therapy
Association (AOTA), 2002. Occupational
therapy practice framework: Domain and
process. Am. J. Occup. Ther. 56, 609–639.
American Occupational Therapy
Association (AOTA), 2008. Occupational
therapy practice framework: Domain and
process. Am. J. Occup. Ther. 62, 625–683.
Baum, C., Christiansen, C., 2005. Person-
Environment-Occupation-Performance:
An occupation-based framework
for practice. In: Christiansen, C.H.,
Baum, C.M., Bass-Haugen, J. (Eds.),
Occupational therapy: Performance,
participation, and well-being, third ed.
Slack, Thorofare, NJ, pp. 243–259.
Brown, C.E., 2009. Ecological models in
occupational therapy. In: Crepeau, E.B.,
Cohn, E.S., Boyt Schell, B.A. (Eds.),
Willard & Spackman's occupational
therapy, eleventh ed. Lippincott Williams &
Wilkins, Baltimore, MD, pp. 435–445.
Bruner, J., 1989. Acts of meaning. Harvard
University Press, Cambridge, MA.

Christiansen, C., 1991. Occupational therapy: Intervention for life performance. In: Christiansen, C., Baum, C. (Eds.), Occupational therapy: Overcoming human performance deficits. Slack, Thorofare, NJ, pp. 3–43.

Christiansen, C., Baum, C., 1991. Occupational therapy: Overcoming human performance deficits. Slack, Thorofare, NJ.

Christiansen, C., Baum, C., 1997a. Person-Environment-Occupational Performance: A conceptual model for practice. In: Christiansen, C., Baum, C. (Eds.), Occupational therapy: Enabling function and well-being, second ed. Slack, Thorofare, NJ, pp. 47–70.

Christiansen, C., Baum, C., 1997b. Understanding occupation: Definitions and concepts. In: Christiansen, C., Baum, C. (Eds.), Occupational therapy: Enabling function and well-being, second ed. Slack, Thorofare, NJ, pp. 3–25.

Christiansen, C., Baum, C., 2005. The complexity of occupation. In: Christiansen, C.H., Baum, C.M. Bass-Haugen, J. (Eds.), Occupational therapy: Performance, participation, and well-being. Slack, Thorofare, NJ, pp. 3–17.

Christiansen, C.H., Baum, C.M., Bass-Haugen, J. (Eds.), 2005. Occupational therapy: Performance, participation, and well-being, third ed. Slack, Thorofare, NJ.

Dunn, W., 2007. Ecology of Human Performance Model. In: Dunbar, S.B. (Ed.), Occupational therapy models for intervention with children and families. Slack, Thorofare, NJ, pp. 127–155.

Dunn, W., Brown, C., McGuigan, A., 1994. The ecology of human performance: A framework for considering the effect of context. Am. J. Occup. Ther. 48(7), 595–607.

Dunn, W., Brown, C., Youngstrom, M.J., 2003. Ecological model of occupation. In: Kramer, P., Hinojosa, J., Royeen, C.B. (Eds.), Perspectives in human occupation: participation in life. Lippincott Williams & Wilkins, Baltimore, MA, pp. 222–263.

Gibson, J.J., 1986. An ecological approach to visual perception. Erlbaum, Hilldale, NJ.

Law, M., Cooper, B., Strong, S., Stewart, D., Rigby, P., Letts, L., 1996. The Person-Environment-Occupation Model: A transactive approach to occupational performance. Can. J. Occup. Ther. 63 (1), 9–23.

Lawton, M.P., 1982. Competence, environmental press, and the adaption of older people. In: Lawton, M.P., Windley, P.G., Byerts, T.O. (Eds.), Aging and the environment. Springer, New York, pp. 33–59.

Murray, H.A., 1938. Explorations in personality. Oxford, New York.

Nelson, D., 1988. Occupation: Form and performance. Am. J. Occup. Ther. 42, 633–641.

Reed, K., 2005. An annotated history of the concepts used in occupational therapy. In: Christiansen, C.H., Baum, C.M., Bass-Haugen, J. (Eds.), Occupational therapy: Performance, participation, and well-being, third ed. Slack, Thorofare, NJ, pp. 567–626.

# Canadian model of occupational performance and engagement

**5**

## CHAPTER CONTENTS

The Canadian Model of Occupational Performance and Engagement (CMOP-E) is one of the three models presented within the larger text on enabling occupation by the Canadian Association of Occupational Therapists. In this chapter, CMOP-E is presented along with two other models, the Canadian Practice Process Framework (CPPF), and the Canadian Model of Client-Centred Enablement (CMCE). Together, these three models present a relatively comprehensive view of the formal position on occupational therapy theory and practice of the Canadian Association of Occupational Therapists.

## MAJOR CONCEPTS AND DEFINITIONS OF TERMS

As with the three models presented in the previous chapter, the Canadian Model of Occupational Performance and Engagement (CMOP-E) aims to make explicit the relationship between person, environment and occupation. It is based on the assumption that occupation, the domain of concern for occupational therapists, is the "bridge that connects person and environment" (p. 23). The model is presented within a larger text entitled *Enabling Occupation II: Advancing an Occupational Therapy Vision for Health, Well-being and Justice through Occupation* (Townsend & Polatajko, 2007). Consequently, many of the assumptions that underpin the model are embedded within the larger text.

117

© 2011 Elsevier Ltd.
DOI: 10.1016/B978-0-7234-3494-8.00005-X

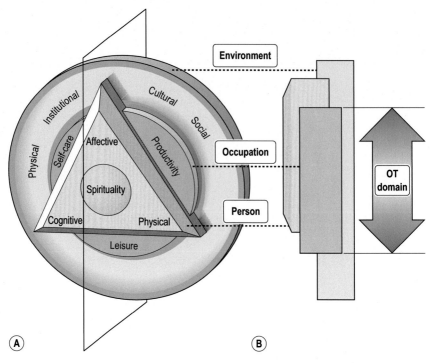

**FIG 5.1    The Canadian Model of Occupational Performance and Engagement (CMOP-E).** *From Elizabeth A. Townsend & Helene J. Polatajko, Enabling occupation II: Advancing an occupational therapy vision for health, well-being and justice through occupation, 2007. Reprinted with the permission of CAOT Publications ACE, Ottawa, Ontario, Canada.*

The three main components of the model are person, occupation and environment. With reference to the diagram (Figure 5.1), these three components were described by Polatajko et al. (2007, p. 23) as follows:

*The* person, *depicted as a triangle at the centre of the model, is portrayed as having three performance components – cognitive, affective, and physical – with spirituality at the core. The model depicts the person embedded within the* environment *to indicate that each individual lives within a unique environmental context – cultural, institutional, physical and social – which affords occupational possibilities.* Occupation *is depicted as the bridge that connects person and environment indicating that individuals act on the environment through occupation. Although the 1997 publication of* Enabling Occupation *indicated that occupation can be classified in numerous ways, the CMOP identified three occupational purposes: self-care, productivity and leisure.*

This description shows that occupation is conceptualized as the agent through which person and occupation interact; portrayed as a bridge. This metaphor conjures the image of person and environment being two distinct entities that are connected through occupation, in the same way that two sides of a river are linked by a bridge. This conceptualization of person and environment as separate entities is similar to the understanding of person and environment in the PEOP model, but differs from the Person-Environment-Occupation model (Law et al., 1996) and Ecology of Human Performance (Dunn et al., 1994), reviewed in the previous chapter, with their transactive or ecological understandings of the relationship between person and environment.

Townsend and Polatajko (2007) presented six basic assumptions that underpin the model. The first two assumptions are based on the work of early occupational therapy writers such as Dunton and Howland and proposed that: (1) humans are occupational beings; and (2) occupation has therapeutic potential. The next three assumptions are that occupation: (3) affects health and well-being; (4) organizes time and brings structure to living; and (5) brings meaning to life through the combination of cultural and individual influences on the creation of meaning. The final assumption is that: (6) occupations are idiosyncratic, in that the specific occupations that a person might engage in will vary from person to person. The authors also clarified that this final assumption qualifies the earlier assumption that occupation affects health and well-being, in that this influence is not always positive; for example, occupations such as drug taking and vandalism can have a negative influence on the person or others.

In *Enabling Occupation II*, occupation was presented as the domain of concern of occupational therapy and an earlier definition of occupation was retained for this edition. Occupation was defined as "groups of activities and tasks of everyday life, named, organized, and given value and meaning by individuals and a culture. Occupation is everything people do to occupy themselves, including looking after themselves (self-care), enjoying life (leisure), and contributing to the social and economic fabric of their communities (productivity)" (CAOT, 1997, cited in Polatajko et al., 2007, p. 17.). Polatajko et al. emphasized that this definition, which would be consistent with most current occupational therapy understandings of occupation, represents a broader concept of the term than both the profession's earlier notion of "occupying the invalid" (p. 17) and the general public's association of occupation with vocation and the means of earning a living. Current occupational therapy notions of occupation refer to all forms of human action that are grouped and have meaning for individuals and cultures. The influence of the occupational performance model on CMOP-E is clear in its classification of the purpose of occupation into the three categories of self-care, productivity and leisure, although this definition of productivity could be seen as relatively broad in that it explicitly refers to the "social and economic fabric" of communities. It is also evident through the term performance components.

As the name suggests, the CMOP-E is a model of *occupational performance*, which is defined as "the dynamic interaction of person, occupation and environment" (Polatajko et al., 2007, p. 23). As the authors explained, the construct of occupational performance is not made explicit in the model but is foundational to and embedded within the model. To use the metaphor we introduced earlier, it is like a window through which one might look rather than a perspective in which the process of looking through the window is described. In the first approach, the window frames what you see but might not be a feature of what you are aware of or describe.

# OCCUPATIONAL ENGAGEMENT AND CLIENT-CENTRED PRACTICE

The CMOP-E proposes that occupational therapy practice requires both enablement and client-centred practice. While the concept of occupational performance remains implicit in the model during its development from the Canadian Model of Occupational Performance (CMOP) (CAOT, 1997) to the CMOP-E (Polatajko et al., 2007), the authors also emphasized that the newer version of this model is not restricted to a focus on occupational performance but also encompasses the concept of *occupational engagement*. In explaining this difference, Polatajko et al. (2007) provided a story about a father and son who participated in marathons together. Their first run together occurred because one of the son's classmates became paralyzed and the school organized a charity run to raise money. The son expressed a strong desire to participate. This event was the start of an occupation that father and son shared for more than four decades. The father ran, pushing his son, severely disabled from birth and only able to communicate using assistive technology operated by his head, in a wheelchair. Over the years they completed a number of marathons, 212 triathlons (in which the son sat in a dinghy and was pulled by the father while he swam) and four ironman events together. These activities had meaning for both of them. After the initial charity run, the son had commented to the father how much he had enjoyed the event because he "didn't feel disabled" (Polatajko et al., 2007, p. 25).This, in turn, motivated the father to pursue subsequent opportunities to participate in the activity together. The "awesome feeling" he gets seeing his son smile is the reason the father does these events (p. 25). The authors used this story to illustrate that occupational performance is a more limited concept than occupational engagement, in that the son did not perform the occupation but engaged in it fully.

This story also illustrates the importance of the second major proposition in *Enabling Occupation II*; that *enablement through occupation* is the current core of occupational therapy. The authors proposed that this focus contrasted with the initial concern of the profession of "the provision of diversional activity" and with the following period in which attention centred on "the use of therapeutic activity" (Polatajko et al., 2007, p. 15). Townsend et al. (2007) reminded readers that enabling occupation had been defined in 1997 as "enabling people to choose, organize, and perform those occupations they find useful and meaningful in their environment" (p. 89). At the time this definition was originally published, choosing and organizing would probably have been considered tasks required to prepare for occupational performance. The newer definition of occupational therapy is based on the assertion that occupational therapists enable through occupation (Townsend et al., 2007). It reads:

> Occupational therapy is the art and science of enabling engagement in everyday living, though occupation; of enabling people to perform the occupations that foster health and well-being; and of enabling a just and inclusive society so that all people may participate to their potential in the daily occupations of life. (p. 89)

The dictionary definition provided by Townsend et al. (2007) for the word *enable* refers to concepts of giving power, strengthening, providing with the ability or means to do something and with the means to do or be something, and making something possible. The definition of occupational therapy provided by the authors emphasizes three types of undertaking that are enabled: (a) people's engagement in everyday life; (b) their performance of occupation; and (c) the development of a just society in which people can participate. For an occupational therapist to enable all three of these outcomes, their practice would need to be aimed at both personal and societal levels.

In recognition of the need to target both personal and societal levels, Townsend et al. (2007) identified six "categories of client" (p. 96) – individuals, families, groups, communities, organizations (including e.g. agencies, clubs and associations, and other government, corporate or non-government organizations) and populations. The authors stated that these categories evolved from four categories presented in the 1997 edition and this expanded view represents a practice that goes beyond working with individuals and might focus on the environment at the levels of client communities, organizations and populations. Detailed definitions of each of these client groups are provided on page 97 of *Enabling Occupation II*.

*Client-centred practice* is also fundamental to CMOP-E. Townsend et al. (2007) commented that client-centred practice means "focusing on client goals and projected outcomes" (p. 98) and pointed out that the following definition, provided in the 1997 edition of *Enabling Occupation*, had concepts of client-centred practice embedded within it. "Enabling is the basis of occupational therapy's client-centred practice and a foundation for client empowerment and justice" (cited in 2007, p. 99). The assumption at the core of both enablement and client-centred practice is that occupational therapy involves "collaborating with people – rather than doing things to or for them" (p. 98). This statement needs to be understood in contrast to a biomedical approach in which 'patients' were primarily expected to be passive recipients of care or curative methods, rather than active participants in the process. Therefore, there might be things that client-centred and enabling occupational therapists *do for* people, such as advocate on their behalf for certain outcomes. However, these do not conjure the image of the passive patient.

Townsend et al. (2007) also noted that there has been a burgeoning of occupational therapy research around the notion of client-centred practice, which has not always "specifi[ed] the connection to enablement" (p. 99). However, the CMOP-E appears to assume a mutual relationship between the two concepts. This is evidenced in the statement, "In occupational therapy, client-centred practice delimits the definition of enablement; conversely enablement delimits the definition of client-centred practice" (Townsend et al., 2007, p. 99). The authors also stated that the challenges to client-centred practice are similar to those of enablement in that they can be encountered at the levels of the client and/or therapist and the broader systems surrounding them. Examples include the client's culture and level of education, the therapist's capacity to share power and recognize client expertise, and the management philosophies and resource distribution of the broader system.

CMOP-E specifies the domain of concern of occupational therapy by identifying the profession's interest in person, environment and occupation, whereby it is through occupation that persons act on the environment. Enablement and client-centred practice are the processes through which occupational therapists facilitate occupational performance and engagement.

As the CMOP-E does not specify this process of enablement, the Canadian Model of Client-Centred Enablement (CMCE) was developed. In the next section, both the Canadian Practice Process Framework and the Canadian Model of Client-Centred Enablement are discussed, to facilitate an understanding of the practice of occupational therapy using the CMOP-E.

## CANADIAN PRACTICE PROCESS FRAMEWORK AND CANADIAN MODEL OF CLIENT-CENTRED ENABLEMENT (CMCE)

In this section, two processes are presented together as they both provide more detailed guidance for the practice of occupational therapy when using the CMOP-E. Each focuses on a different aspect of the occupational therapy process. The Canadian Practice Process Framework (CPPF) aims to make explicit the action points in the broader occupational therapy process, which occurs with the client within a broader societal and practice context. The Canadian Model of Client-Centred Enablement (CMCE) focuses on the encounter between occupational therapist and client (also called the therapeutic relationship in the broader occupational therapy literature) and aims to make explicit the process of enabling occupation in a client-centred way.

## CANADIAN PRACTICE PROCESS FRAMEWORK (CPPF)

Craik et al. (2007) stated that the CPPF for occupational therapy is "a process framework for evidence-based, client-centred occupational enablement" (p. 233). This framework seems to have been developed in response to the feedback obtained regarding the Occupational Performance Process Model (OPPM), published by Fearing et al. (1997), which was seen to be "useful to guide individualized practice" (pp. 231–232) but not designed for nor appropriate to practice with "community, organization, or population clients" (p. 232). In contrast, Craik et al. proposed that the CPPF can be used with all six categories of client discussed earlier in relation to enablement. The diagrammatic representation of the CPPF is presented in Figure 5.2.

As Craik et al. (2007) stated, "The CPPF guides the therapist through a process of occupation-based, evidence-based, and client-centred practice, which is directed towards enabling change in occupational performance and engagement. By utilizing the CPPF, an occupational therapist would identify eight key actions in enabling any type of client to reach occupational goals." (p. 234.) These key action points include the commencement and conclusion of the process (called enter/initiate and conclude/exit) and six other general process points. These general points are: set the stage; assess/evaluate; agree on objectives, plans; implement plan; monitor/modify; and evaluate outcome.

As the diagram shows, while the six steps between entering and exiting the process are connected by solid arrows, indicating the general process of professional action, dotted arrows also indicate alternate paths. For example, a service that only provides assessment might follow a path through the first three action points and then proceed straight to the exit point, having only made recommendations. Similarly, one cycle through the pathway might not be sufficient to address the occupational issues identified, or the goals and

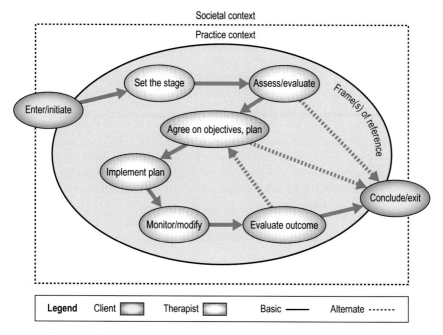

**FIG 5.2** The Canadian Practice Process Framework (CPPF). *From Elizabeth A. Townsend & Helene J. Polatajko, Enabling occupation II: Advancing an occupational therapy vision for health, well-being and justice through occupation, 2007. Reprinted with the permission of CAOT Publications ACE, Ottawa, Ontario, Canada.*

desired outcomes might change as a result of the changes made during the first cycle through the pathway. Therefore, repeated cycles might be required. The diagram indicates that the whole process occurs within the broader societal and practice context. These two entities are separated by dotted lines to denote their interrelatedness. In addition, the six action points between entering and exiting the process occur in the context of a frame or frames of reference. This circle "indicates the professional knowledge the therapist brings to the process" (p. 235), which is "defined within the local practice and daily living context" (p. 251) and shaped by the broader societal context.

The first two action points in the CPPF are *enter/initiate* and *set the scene*. In these early steps, once the 'client' has been defined using one of the six categories of client (individual, family, group, organization, community or population), there is the need to establish a collaborative relationship and engage in processes such as rapport building, setting ground-rules, clarifying expectations and facilitating the client's preparedness to proceed. Next follows *assessment* of "occupational status, dreams, and potential for change", including analysis of "spirituality, person, and environmental influences on occupations" (p. 251). The fourth action point is to *agree on objectives and plans*. Negotiating an agreement requires a collaborative decision-making process and involves "reflecting upon the client's occupational challenges, the priority occupational issues, and assessment/evaluation findings, including data on occupations and the personal and environmental factors influencing occupational engagement" (p. 258). The next three action points are typically included in descriptions of professional practice. These are to *implement the plan, monitor and modify* it as necessary and *evaluate* the outcome. The encounter is then concluded and the client exits. The flexibility of the path occurs when there is a change to the plan on the basis of the evaluation of the outcome or the client exits after some of the earlier action points.

Throughout the process, the importance of "client participation and power sharing as much as possible" (p. 251) is emphasized. The overall aim in following this process is to "enable the client to pursue occupational performance or engagement goals" (p. 234) and, therefore, goal attainment is the desired outcome of the process. Its relationship to the other two models is made explicit in the following statement, "This outcome [goal attainment] will be achieved by effective application of the CMOP-E, focused on occupation and using key enablement skills [of the CMCE]: adapt, advocate, coach, collaborate, consult, coordinate, design/build, educate, engage, and specialize" (p. 234). As each of the action points is discussed, the specific enablement skills from the CMCE relevant to that action point are presented.

## CANADIAN MODEL OF CLIENT-CENTRED ENABLEMENT (CMCE)

While the CPPF outlines the action points within the occupational therapy process, the CMCE details the nature of the encounter between client and occupational therapist. Both are necessary for client-centred occupational therapy practice.

The CMCE was described as "a visual metaphor for client-centred enablement" and the stated purpose of client-centred enablement is to "advance a vision of health, well-being, and justice through occupation" (Townsend et al. (2007), p. 109). Its diagrammatic representation is presented in Figure 5.3.

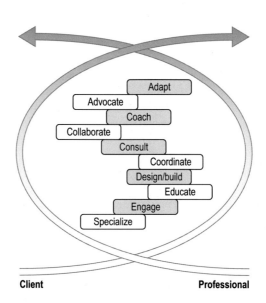

**FIG 5.3**   The Canadian Model of Client-Centred Enablement. *From Elizabeth A. Townsend & Helene J. Polatajko, Enabling occupation II: Advancing an occupational therapy vision for health, well-being and justice through occupation, 2007. Reprinted with the permission of CAOT Publications ACE, Ottawa, Ontario, Canada.*

As the diagram shows, the CMCE represents the relationship between client and professional as two asymmetrical, curved lines that intersect in two places and enclose 10 alphabetically ordered verbs that identify the skills necessary for enablement (called enablement skills). Townsend et al. (2007) stated that the CMCE is based on two premises: "that enablement is occupational therapists' core competency" and that "client-centred enablement is based on enablement foundations and employs enablement skills in a collaborative relationship with clients [of all six categories]" (p. 109). Central to the CMCE are enablement foundations and enablement skills. Each is described briefly.

Townsend et al. (2007) listed six client-centred, occupation-based *enablement foundations*. These are: choice, risk, responsibility; client participation; visions of possibility; change; justice; and power-sharing. As they stated, "enablement foundations are the interests, values, beliefs, ideas, concepts, critical perspectives, and concerns that shape enablement reasoning and priorities" (p. 100). These enablement foundations appear to have been underpinned by a concern for equality of opportunity and the awareness that people with disabilities are marginalized in many societies and have reduced opportunities to access socially valued resources and roles. Each foundation is discussed.

- In discussing *choice, risk and responsibility*, the authors stressed that occupational therapists have an ethical obligation to respect "client views, experience, interests, and safety" (p. 100) as well as their right to make choices and live with risk.
- *Client participation* is presented as pertaining to citizenship and the right of people to participate in their societies and communities. They stated that clients are "entitled to participate in making decisions about occupational therapy, other services, and their lives" (p. 101).
- The term *visions of possibility* (p. 102) is used to refer to "*what might be* or even *what could be*" (p. 103, italics in original), rather than being constrained by how things are at the time. Townsend et al. proposed that occupational therapists can facilitate their clients to "imagine a life that may not be expected of them and that they may not have expected" (p. 102).
- While the fourth enablement foundation is labelled *change*, it also includes the goal of preventing change, if this is appropriate to the client. As the authors explained, "change might be directed to enable clients to (a) develop through occupational transitions across the lifecourse, (b) maintain occupational engagement, health and well-being, (c) restore occupational potential and performance, or (d) prevent occupational losses and deprivation, occupational alienation, or other forms of occupational injustice" (p. 103).
- Townsend et al. identified four aspects of a *justice* perspective on enabling. These related to recognizing injustices that are systematically encountered by various groups in society, accepting people as they are, advocating for people and their rights to participate equally in society, and noticing when we or others assume that people need to change or improve some aspect of themselves to be more acceptable (as distinct from when a client might identify the goal to change).

- The authors proposed that *power-sharing* is central to client-centred collaboration and this requires an explicit and conscious process. They stated, "successful, collaborative power-sharing involves genuine interest, acknowledgement, empathy, altruism, trust, and creative communication" (p. 107).

These enablement foundations are central to creating client-centred enablement and underpin the CMCE. Within the CMCE, 10 *enablement skills* are also identified. These are (presented in alphabetical order to assist memory): adapt, advocate, coach, collaborate, consult, coordinate, design/build, educate, engage, and specialize. According to the authors, these ten skills were selected because they appeared to "capture the essence of occupational therapy" (p. 112) when field testing the list. However, they were also presented with other generic occupational therapy enablement skills, categorized as process, professional and scholarship skills (see Table 5.1 for the full list).

Townsend et al. (2007) outlined eight principles that underlie the use of enablement skills across the diversity of occupational therapy practice. These are:

1. Occupational therapists typically employ a combination of enablement skills (rather than just one) in any particular situation
2. Different enablement skills might be required as the situation unfolds in response to needs of client in context.
3. While occupational therapists strive for mutual and reciprocal collaboration, the specific nature of that collaboration will vary across different clients.
4. Depending on their interest, talents and experiences, individual occupational therapists develop a unique range of enablement skills. Different skills might also be more effective or appropriate in different settings.
5. Enablement skills can be visible or invisible to others. At times, client empowerment might increase with minimal awareness of the professional's contribution to the process. At other times, it might be important for professionals to be able to articulate their enablement skills to prevent them from being undervalued.
6. Enablement skills should be based on the best available evidence from a variety of sources including client experience.

Table 5.1    *Generic skills that underpin enablement*

| Process skills | Analyze, Assess, Critique, Empathize, Evaluate, Examine, Implement, Intervene, Investigate, Plan, Reflect |
|---|---|
| Professional skills | Comply with ethical and moral codes, Comply with professional regulatory requirements, Document practice |
| Scholarship skills | Use evidence, Evaluate programs and services, Generate and disseminate knowledge, Transfer knowledge |

7. Occupational therapists have a responsibility to use their enablement skills of *educate* with students and other staff.
8. Enablement skills are used across the eight action points of the CPPF and throughout the entire practice process.

Townsend et al. (2007) provided a one to two page discussion of each of the 10 enablement skills. However, they stated that these summaries "are intended to be introductory, not comprehensive. The brief outlines are intended to stimulate interest to describe and critically reflect on occupational therapy's core competency in client-centred enablement" (p. 116). This statement is important to keep in mind when reviewing the descriptions provided here, which aim to provide only a very brief overview of the enablement skills. Each of the enablement skills is specifically linked to the first five of the seven *competency roles* published by the Canadian Association of Occupational Therapists. These five are: change agent, communicator, collaborator, expert in enabling occupation, practice manager, with practice scholar and profession being roles that underlie all of the enablement skills.

- Adapt: This enablement skill is linked to the role of change agent. The discussion of adapting is mainly targeted towards altering occupations (e.g. breaking down tasks to create just-right challenges) but adapting could equally be applied to altering the environment or selecting a different environment to enable occupation. The related enablement skills identified are synthesizing, occupational analyses and proposing recommendations for adaptations.
- Advocate: This skill is also linked to the role of change agent. It might include raising awareness in others of problem issues and promoting the need for these issues to be addressed by those who have the power to change them, challenging others to think differently about an issue, and championing a cause. Related enablement skills are listed as forming alliances and partnerships and developing lobby groups with others.
- Coach: The related competency roles are collaborator and communicator. The general aim of coaching in occupational therapy is to "encourage clients to reflect and discover their own motivations in their desired occupations" (p. 119). This could be done through conversations with clients about occupation. In some instances, these may result in clients' occupational engagement. Related enablement skills include "engaging others in occupations, and listening to client voices, meanings, and mental models" and "engaging people in self-assessment of their strengths, resources, challenges, and desired goals" (p. 119).
- Collaborate: Townsend et al. stated that this is "arguably the key enablement skill for power-sharing in client-centred practice" (p. 119, emphasis in original) and emphasized that collaboration involves working *with* people rather than doing things to or for them. As would be expected, it is associated with the collaborator competency role. Examples of the many related enablement skills are seeking multiple perspectives, promoting alliances and facilitating the resolution of differences through active negotiation.
- Consult: This key enablement skill is essential to the role of expert in enabling occupation. It is required for practice with clients and in management, education and research. It may replace direct service

in specific situations and require occupational therapists to gather information, synthesize it into an in-depth understanding of the situation or issue and involve actions such as giving advice, making recommendations and advocating for change. Related enablement skills "are brainstorming options [and] conferring or holding counsel as a basis for advising others" (p. 121).

- Coordinate: This enablement skill is seen as essential to the leadership competency role of practice manager. As the authors stated, "coordination draws on occupational therapists' strong integration skills in which therapists synthesize, analyse, and act on the broad range of information on occupations, and the personal and environmental influences" (p. 122). They coordinate information, people, services and organizations and may be acting in direct service and case coordination roles, as well as management roles. Related enablement skills are to be able to elicit multiple perspectives and reframe differences in order to find a common ground for collaboration. It may require occupational therapists to "educate those involved, and to facilitate, mediate, or actively negotiate networking, links, and resolutions. Also related are skills to integrate, synthesize, organise, lead, and supervise." (p. 123.)

- Design/build: The competency role related to this enablement skill is change agent. Occupational therapists might design and build assistive technology or orthotics or use these skills to adapt environments and design and implement programs and services. Townsend et al. noted that "occupational therapists are known for conceiving, creating, designing, redesigning, rebuilding, and in some cases fabricating, constructing, or manufacturing products and environmental adaptations" (p. 123). In connection to related enablement skills they wrote that these skills "are connected with enablement skills to design a coaching strategy, to adapt environments, to advocate for social change, to collaborate with stakeholders, to coordinate multiple efforts across sectors, to educate communities about universal and inclusive design, and to engage clients in the design and building of environments that enable them to live in health, well-being and justice" (p. 123).

- Educate: This enablement skill is also linked to the competency role of change agent. The description of this skill is broader than just the provision of information that is often associated with client education. Instead, the skill of educating is linked to an understanding of educational philosophy and teaching and learning principles. In illustrating their proposition that occupational therapists "use occupations for *learning through doing*", Townsend et al. stated, "Occupational therapists are particularly skilled in the educational use of simulated occupations in hospitals or other settings designed to offer therapy apart from the natural environment… Where occupational therapy facilities have been created, client education may involve demonstrating or practising simulated occupations before clients transfer their learning to their own home, work, or other environments. Clients… learn through doing with instruction in performing or organizing routines of occupations, or in adapting the environment" (p. 124). The related enablement skills listed are facilitating rote, repetitive and instrumental learning as well as "facilitating, guiding, prompting, listening, reflecting, encouraging, and supporting" (p. 125).

- Engage: The skill of engaging is associated with the competency role of expert in enabling occupation. Central to client-centred practice is the ability to engage clients actively in occupation and the ICF defines participation as engagement in valued social roles. Regarding related enablement skills, Townsend et al. stated, "occupational therapists may need to combine engagement skills with collaboration skills in dispute resolution, mediation, and coordination skills to bring together diverse perspectives and competing interests" (p. 127).
- Specialize: This enablement skill is seen as a composite of skills that contribute to the competency role of expert in enabling occupation. In the process of specializing, occupational therapists develop a range of skills. Examples could include therapeutic touch and positioning, the use of particular sensory-motor techniques, and psychosocial rehabilitation techniques. In the process of specializing, occupational therapists require both skills development and an understanding of the relevant specialized theoretical and philosophical perspectives and knowledge bases. The challenge when specializing is to remain client-centred and to ensure that "clients understand, agree with, and participate, as they are able and wish to, in specialized approaches" (p. 127). There are no related enabling skills listed, possibly because specialization is already considered to be a composite of skills.

Enablement foundations and skills are used within the context of a client-centred relationship. Within the CMCE, the purpose of the relationship between client and occupational therapy professional is to enable "individual and social change" through occupation (p. 109). This change occurs in both an individual's occupational performance and engagement and the "social structures that influence engagement in everyday life" (p. 109).

With reference to the CMCE diagram, Townsend et al. (2007) stated:

> A central feature of the CMCE is the two asymmetrical, curved lines. They represent the dynamism, changeability, variability, risk-taking, and power differences present in the client-professional relationship. The asymmetrical curve suggests the possibility of diverse forms of collaboration. The evolving nature of client-professional collaboration means that they will not be symmetrical, straightforward, static, standardized, predictable, or prescriptive. (p. 109)

The points at which the two lines cross represent the entry and exit points in the occupational therapy process outlined in the CPPF and the presence of boundaries in the relationship. The 10 enablement skills discussed lie within the space bounded by the two lines and guide occupational therapy practice through all of the eight action points. In the CMCE, the entry and exit points can be used to frame a single interaction or the beginning and end of the entire occupational therapy process. "The boundaries of enablement will vary with the referral or contract, service conditions, the physical environment, and the socio-cultural, economic, political, and institutional context" (p. 111). While power imbalances are an inherent feature of professional–client relationships, the sharing of power is central to the client-centred approach upon which the CMCE is based.

In summary, the three practice models/frameworks presented in this chapter are designed to be used in combination. The CMOP-E provides the overall structure for conceptualizing occupational performance and engagement and the work of occupational therapists. The CPPF provides details about the generic process used by occupational therapists when working with clients, and the CMCE provides an action framework within which to conceptualize *how* occupational therapists work with their clients.

## HISTORICAL DESCRIPTION OF THE MODEL'S DEVELOPMENT

The Canadian health system appears to have a greater degree of national integration and standardization than many other Western countries. Consistent with this trend, the Canadian Association of Occupational Therapists (CAOT) has tended to publish position statements and theoretical frameworks that have aimed to guide occupational therapists across that nation in a more integrated way than any other Western country. This is not to suggest that the occupational therapy associations in other countries have not assembled national guidelines (the AOTA's OTPF would be an example), but to place into a broader context the CMOP-E authors' claim that the model is the "graphic representation of the Canadian perspective on occupation, or more specifically on occupational performance" (Polatajko et al. 2007, p. 27).

The CMOP-E was published as the CMOP in the first edition of *Enabling Occupation* (CAOT, 1997). According to Polatajko et al. (2007), CMOP was "updated from the Occupational Performance Model (OPM) that was presented in the 1991 CAOT guidelines" (p. 23). As has been emphasized throughout this book, the concept of occupational performance was a major focus of occupational therapy theorists writing in the 1990s. While occupational performance is an important concept in many occupational therapy models, the authors of *Enabling Occupation II* were careful to explain the difference between the CMOP and the CMOP-E by discussing the distinction between occupational performance and occupational engagement. They proposed that the latter, broader concept is "congruent" with current occupational therapy concerns (p. 24). Consistent with the periods in occupational therapy's history described by Reed (2005) and Kielhofner (2009), the authors of the CMOP and CMOP-E stated that, "early in our history there was strong objection raised to describing our work as occupying people because of [the phrase's] association with ordinary diversion of keeping busy, without the professional value of therapy" (Polatajko et al., 2007, p. 24). They claimed this emphasis might no longer be the case. (This is possibly due to a combination of the broader concepts of health pervading the wider Western health context and the renaissance of occupation that has occurred in occupational therapy.)

CMOP and CMOP-E form part of a long line of documents produced by CAOT. The 1997 edition of *Enabling Occupation* (CAOT, 1997) presented a review of the five major guidelines documents and the Canadian Occupational Performance Measure (COPM) produced by CAOT from 1980 to 1993. The introduction emphasized that all of these documents advocated client-centred practice and a focus on occupational performance. Three documents outlining guidelines for the client-centred practice of occupational therapy were produced in French and English between 1980 and 1987.

The third *guidelines* document recommended the development of an outcome measure. As a result, the COPM was developed. According to CAOT, this assessment tool was based on the OPM presented in the 1983 guidelines. A fourth general guidelines document was published in 1991 and guidelines relating to client-centred practice in mental health were published in 1993. All of these guidelines were based on the OPM.

To place the development of the CMOP and CMOP-E within the context of these documents is important as both models have developed in conjunction with the progression from ideas in the Occupational Performance Model (with its inclusion of the concepts of performance components), through a focus on occupational performance in the CMOP, to the inclusion of the concept of occupational engagement in the CMOP-E. The influence of the earlier Occupational Performance Model on both CMOP and CMOP-E is evident in their concepts and some of their language. For example, the diagram used to represent the CMOP-E (see Figure 5.1) shows the person as having affective, cognitive and physical "performance components" (Polatajko et al., 2007, p. 23).

One of the major changes that occurred between the CMOP and the CMOP-E relates to the definition of the client. This probably reflects the changing nature of occupational therapy practice and the increasing diversity of roles that occupational therapists are undertaking as well as the changing concepts relating to health in the broader society. At the time the CMOP was developed, a main focus of CAOT was the principle of client-centred practice. The visual representation of CMOP showed the person in the centre of the diagram, surrounded by the three areas of occupation and the four aspects of the environment. This kind of approach aimed to emphasize the holistic, *person-centred* nature of the model. Law et al. (1997) stated, "The new Canadian Model of Occupational Performance presents the person as an integrated whole who incorporates spirituality, social and cultural experiences, and observable occupational performance components" (p. 41).

To provide clarification about their understanding of client, the authors wrote, "Clients are individuals who may have occupational problems arising from medical conditions, transitional difficulties, or environmental barriers, or clients can be organizations that influence the occupational performance of particular groups or populations" (p. 50). They also emphasized that the principles underpinning client-centred practice still apply to organizations, etc. as occupational therapists need to collaborate with clients and respect their decisions. More recently, the CMOP-E identified six categories of clients – individuals, families, groups, communities, organizations and populations. What is yet to be clarified is how the diagrammatic representation of this person-centred model that includes affective, cognitive and physical performance components relates to the practice with communities, organizations and populations.

## SUMMARY

CMOP-E is offered as representing the official position of the CAOT. It is a client-centred model that developed out of the occupational performance model tradition that was particularly influential in North America during the 1970s and 1980s. In the diagram, person, environment and occupation, the three major components of the model, are represented as three con-centric layers surrounding an inner core. The individual is placed in the centre of the diagram with a core of spirituality surrounded by cognitive, affective and physical performance components. Three performance areas of self-care, productivity and leisure form the next layer of occupation. Physical, institutional, cultural and social environments form the outer-most layer. Occupation is conceptualized as the bridge between person and environment.

CMOP-E is the second edition of the CMOP. It distinguishes between occupational performance and occupational engagement, in that people can engage in occupation without necessarily performing it. CMOP-E includes a broader definition of the client that uses the six categories of individuals, families, groups, communities, organizations and populations. In *Enabling Occupation II*, three models/frameworks are presented together to guide occu-pational therapists to facilitate occupational performance and engagement in a client-centred way.

See Box 5.1.

---

> **BOX 5.1** The Canadian Model of Occupational Performance and Engagement (CMOP-E) memory aid
>
> What category of client am I working with?
>
> (individual, family, group, community, organization, population)
>
> What are the client's goals and what goal/s does our collaboration have?
>
> What are the client's spiritual (values-based) beliefs and how might they affect occupational performance and engagement?
>
> (individual spirituality, the spiritual culture of a community/population, the ethical position of the organization)
>
> - What occupations have meaning for the client?
>
> - How would the client's self-identity/purpose change if they were no longer able to perform or engage in those occupations?
>
> What is the status of the client's performance components (affective, cognitive & physical) and how might they affect occupational performance and engagement?
>
> What are the physical, institutional, cultural and social aspects of the environment surrounding the client and how might they affect the client's occupational performance and engagement?
>
> How does the client interact with the environment through occupation?
>
> (In what ways does occupation form a bridge between the person and the environment?)
>
> - Occupations the client performs to fulfil social roles
>
> - Occupations that give the client access to environmental resources
>
> Which enablement skills do I need to use in this situation?
>
> (Adapt, Advocate, Coach, Collaborate, Consult, Coordinate, Design/Build, Educate, Engage, Specialize)

Canadian model of occupational performance and engagement

# CONCLUSION

In this chapter we examined the CMOP-E, originally published as the CMOP. The reason for the name change was the development in thinking from an emphasis on occupational performance alone to occupational performance and engagement. The rationale for this changed emphasis is that people can be engaged in occupation without performing it.

This model emphasizes the societal aspects of occupational performance and engagement in that it recognizes that, within society, people might have differing opportunities for engagement in and performance of occupation. This awareness of inequity and the barriers to occupation that disabled people often face is central to the model and expressed through the concept of justice. Because of this concern, occupational therapists can take on roles such as advocacy that are additional to traditional concepts of occupational therapy practice.

In this chapter, we presented not only the CMOP-E but also the CPPF and the CMCE. In combination, the three models aim to guide client-centred practice that focuses on promoting a just approach to occupational performance and enablement. In the chapter that follows, the Model of Human Occupation is presented. That is the model of practice that has influenced occupational theory and practice for the longest and most sustained period of time. As with the CMOP-E, it has important features of the model that are unique to that particular model.

## MAJOR WORKS

Canadian Association of Occupational Therapists, 1997. Enabling occupation: An occupational therapy perspective. CAOT Publications ACE, Ottawa, ON.

Canadian Association of Occupational Therapists, 2002. Enabling occupation: An occupational therapy perspective.

(Revised edition). CAOT Publications ACE, Ottawa, ON.

Townsend, E.A., Polatajko, H.J. (Eds.), 2007. Enabling occupation II: Advancing an occupational therapy vision for health, well-being and justice through occupation. CAOT Publications ACE, Ottawa, ON.

## REFERENCES

Canadian Association of Occupational Therapists, 1997. Enabling occupation: An occupational therapy perspective. CAOT Publications ACE, Ottawa, ON.

Craik, J., Davis, J., Polatajko, H., 2007. Introducing the Canadian Practice Process Framework (CPPF): Amplifying the context. In: Townsend, E.A., Polatajko, H.J. (Eds.), Enabling occupation II: Advancing an occupational therapy vision for health, well-being, and justice through occupation. CAOT Publications ACE, Ottawa, ON, pp. 229–246.

Dunn, W., Brown, C., McGuigan, A., 1994. The ecology of human performance: A framework for considering the effect of context. Am. J. Occup. Ther. 48(7), 595–607.

Fearing, V.G., Law, M., Clark, M., 1997. An occupational performance process model: Fostering client and therapist alliances. Can. J. Occup. Ther. 64 (1), 7–15.

Kielhofner, G., 2009. Conceptual foundations of occupational therapy practice, fourth ed. F.A. Davis, Philadelphia, PA.

Law, M., Cooper, B., Strong, S., Stewart, D., Rigby, P., Letts, L., 1996.

The Person-Environment-Occupation Model: A transactive approach to occupational performance. Can. J. Occup. Ther. 63 (1), 9–23.

Law, M., Polatajko, H., Baptist, S., Townsend, E., 1997. Core concepts in occupational therapy. In: Canadian Association of Occupational Therapists (CAOT) (Eds.), Enabling occupation: An occupational therapy perspective. CAOT Publications ACE, Ottawa, ON, pp. 29–56.

Polatajko, H.J., Davis, J., Stewart, D., et al., 2007. Specifying the domain of concern: Occupation as core. In: Townsend, E.A., Polatajko, H.J. (Eds.), Enabling occupation II: Advancing an occupational therapy vision for health, well-being, and justice through occupation. CAOT Publications ACE, Ottawa, ON, pp. 13–36.

Reed, K., 2005. An annotated history of the concepts used in occupational therapy. In: Christiansen, C.H., Baum, C.M., Bass-Haugen, J. (Eds.), Occupational therapy: Performance, participation, and well-being, third ed. Slack, Thorofare, NJ, pp. 567–626.

Townsend, E.A., Beagan, B., Kumas-Tan, Z., et al., 2007. Enabling: Occupational therapy's core competency. In: Townsend, E.A., Polatajko, H.J. (Eds.), Enabling occupation II: Advancing an occupational therapy vision for health, well-being, and justice through occupation. CAOT Publications ACE, Ottawa, ON, pp. 87–133.

Townsend, E.A., Polatajko, H.J. (Eds.), 2007. Enabling occupation II: Advancing an occupational therapy vision for health, well-being, and justice through occupation. CAOT Publications ACE, Ottawa, ON.

Canadian model of occupational performance and engagement

# Model of human occupation

6

## CHAPTER CONTENTS

The Model of Human Occupation, or MOHO (Kielhofner, 1985, 1995, 2002, 2008) as it is well known, is the longest published model in occupational therapy. It developed out of the occupational behaviour tradition at the University of Southern California, USA. At the time it was first published, the major occupational therapy models available in North America were the occupational performance models. As they primarily focused on physical rehabilitation, MOHO was unique in that it addressed issues relevant to other areas of practice such as mental health and intellectual disability through its detailed description of *volition* and *habituation*. Perhaps owing to its broad scope, MOHO was very influential in both these specific areas as well as more broadly.

## MAIN CONCEPTS AND DEFINITIONS OF TERMS

As the name suggests, the Model of Human Occupation was established to explore, organize and make explicit the concept of human occupation, which was considered the foundation of occupational therapy. The model has undergone substantial changes since its original publications in the early 1980s and many of these changes are detailed in the historical description section of this chapter. This section discusses the major concepts as they were presented in the fourth edition of the major text (Kielhofner, 2008).

© 2011 Elsevier Ltd.
DOI: 10.1016/B978-0-7234-3494-8.00006-1

In the fourth edition, Kielhofner (2008) stated, "The vision for MOHO has been to support practice throughout the world that is occupation-focussed, client-centred, evidence-based, and complementary to practice based on other occupational therapy models and interdisciplinary theories." (p. 1.) In some ways the model is difficult to describe, because it has evolved substantially in its concepts, since the first edition of the text in 1985, whilst keeping its original structural components.

It is difficult to identify the overall purpose of MOHO in its current (and previous) edition as these latest writings have highlighted the model's newest developments and changes, without necessarily making explicit the model's purpose. However, to use the metaphor of the window through which one looks without making the process of looking out the window explicit, it may be that MOHO centres on the processes of occupational adaptation, without stating it overtly. The core concepts of the model were listed as "environmental impact, volition, habituation, performance capacity, participation, performance, skills, occupational identity, and occupational competence" (Kielhofner, 2008, p. 145). Figure 6.1 shows how their relationships are organized, with all of the concepts leading to occupational adaptation. Therefore, *occupational adaptation* might be the overall focus of MOHO.

Figure 6.1 outlines how a person engages in human occupation within the context of the environment and this process results in occupational adaptation. Three concepts are considered to be internal to the person. These are volition, habituation and performance capacity and are concepts that have been associated with MOHO since its origins. Additionally, human occupation is conceptualized as having three dimensions. These are participation, performance and skill. When a person engages in occupation, it creates a change in occupational identity and occupational competence, both of which are conceptualized as the components of occupational adaptation. All of this occurs in the context of an environment that shapes and is shaped by all aspects of the process.

The first aspect of the model that we will describe is the original concepts associated with MOHO – volition, habituation, performance capacity and environment (Figure 6.2). Kielhofner (2008) stated that MOHO aims to provide a framework for conceptualizing how people "select, organize and undertake their occupations" (p. 12). An earlier version of the model described this aim as the parallel concern for how occupation is "motivated, patterned and performed" (Kielhofner, 2002, p. 13). The model attends to each of these

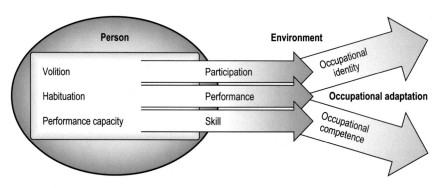

**FIG 6.1** The process of occupational adaptation. *(adapted from Kielhofner, 2008, p. 108)*

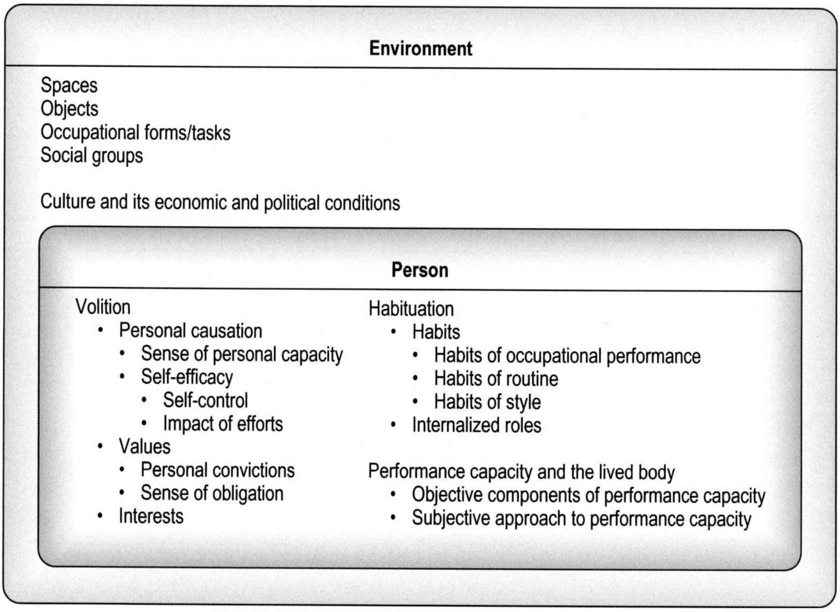

FIG 6.2 The basic concepts of human occupation.

aims through the concepts of volition, habituation and performance capacity, respectively. That is, volition explains why people select occupations, habituation outlines how they organize their occupations and performance capacity attends to the skills and abilities that enable them to perform their occupations. Human occupation is also conceptualized as existing within an environmental context that influences all aspects of occupation. These environments provide opportunities, as well as support, demand and constrain occupation. In discussing environment, the model details physical and social environments and uses the term occupational settings to refer to the overall context surrounding occupation.

## VOLITION

The concept of volition is finely detailed in MOHO. This is one of the unique features of the model, as this level of detail about volition does not occur in any of the other models. The human need to act is presented as pervasive, intense and the basis for occupation. The model uses the term *volition* to refer to this impetus towards action. Kielhofner (2008) defined volition as "a pattern of thoughts and feelings about oneself as an actor in one's world which occurs as one anticipates, chooses, experiences, and interprets what one does" (p. 16). MOHO presents volitional thoughts and feelings as including three components – personal causation, values and interests – and a volitional process that includes a cycle of anticipation, making choices, experience and interpretation. Each of the three components of volition is influenced by this volitional cycle, in which volition affects how people anticipate action, make choices about what action they will engage in, experience action and interpret or give meaning to their actions. Each of these components of volition also comprises other elements.

First, *personal causation* refers to "one's sense of capacity and effectiveness" (Kielhofner, 2008, p. 13). The term personal causation is used in the sense that people can experience themselves as being able to cause or make things happen, that is, to be able to act purposefully in the world and produce outcomes. Personal causation is conceptualized as comprising two elements, a sense of both *personal capacity* and *self-efficacy*. These refer respectively to people's thoughts and feelings about what they are capable of and their sense of what kinds of outcomes they are able to control. It may be that people's sense of personal capacity pertains to something that is within them (but affects how they operate within the world), whereas self-efficacy operates more overtly in their relationships with the world. While people can experience a sense of capacity, they can also encounter incapacity, which "is experienced as difficulty doing the things that matter in one's life" (p. 37).

Self-efficacy requires both self-control and a sense of being able to bring about a desired outcome. It relates to specific spheres of life, in that people might feel they can control outcomes in some areas more than others (Kielhofner, 2008). Experiences contribute to the development of both personal capacity and self-efficacy in that people are more likely to persist or seek out opportunities in situations in which they feel capable or efficacious and to avoid situations that do not provide that kind of feedback or outcome. Often, the sudden or gradual loss of personal capacities leads to a reduced sense of self-efficacy, just as the contexts in which people conduct their lives can enhance or reduce their self-efficacy.

Second, MOHO presents *values* as contributing fundamentally to the volition for action. Values are the "beliefs and commitments" that people develop about "what is good, right, and important to do" (Kielhofner, 2008, p. 39). The values that individuals hold are developed in relation to the broader culture in which they have grown up and live. Kielhofner suggested that, as values are developed from cultural norms, people develop a sense of belonging to the cultural group when acting in ways that are consistent with their values and experience guilt and shame when acting in contravention of those values.

MOHO associates two concepts with values. These are personal convictions and a sense of obligation. Respectively, these link values to the worldviews that people hold and the actions they are likely to take. Kielhofner (2008) defined *personal convictions* as "strongly held views of life that define what matters" (p. 40). Personal convictions are more than what people believe and include their worldviews and perspectives. That is, they are what persons believe to be important. Whereas some aspects of a worldview might be relatively easy to change, personal convictions about what matters are not. MOHO also emphasizes the connection between values and action. Kielhofner (2008) suggested that "values bind people to action" (p. 41) through a *sense of obligation* to act in ways that are consistent with their values. Therefore, self-esteem and sense of self-worth can be reduced when people's ability to perform is not consistent with their values or those of the society (where those societal values matter to them). In addition, where enduring changes to people's capacities occur (which change their ability to act in the world), the need for action and values to be consistent can prompt a process of revising one's values.

The third aspect of volition is *interests*. This concept relates to those things that people find enjoyable or satisfying. As Kielhofner (2008) stated, "interests reveal themselves both as the enjoyment of doing something and as a preference for doing certain things over others" (p. 42). Enjoyment can derive from any constellation of factors including bodily pleasure, fulfilment from intellectual and artistic pleasures, the handling of materials and production of something pleasing, and fellowship with others. Kielhofner associated the attraction individuals might have to particular occupations with the concept of "flow" (Csikszentmihalyi, 1990). In flow experiences, people are engaged deeply in something and often experience a sense of timelessness. Flow experiences result when the demands of the activity or occupation optimally match the capacities of the individual. The implication is that enjoyment (and, therefore, interest) typically increases when individual capacities match activity demands.

Kielhofner also suggested that people develop a unique pattern of interests, which accumulates through experience. People make choices about occupation over time, according to their preferences, and these often develop into a pattern of choices. He suggested that the patterns of interests that people develop are "usually paralleled by a routine in which their interests are at least partially indulged" (p. 44). The concept of a pattern of interests forms a link to the next component of MOHO: habituation.

## HABITUATION

MOHO proposes that the things that people do in their daily lives become routinized and taken for granted through a process of habituation. Habituation is defined as "an internalized readiness to exhibit consistent patterns of behaviour guided by habits and roles and fitted to the characteristics of routine temporal, physical and social environments" (Kielhofner, 2008, p. 52). It serves the purpose of reducing the degree to which decisions about action have to be made consciously.

Habituation is assumed to require cooperation with the environment in order to support people's routine action, in that, a degree of environmental stability is necessary for the development of habitual occupational performance. Using an image with broader application than to humans alone, Kielhofner stated, "The regularity in habituated behaviour depends on the reliability of habitats" (p. 52). The stability of habits relies on temporal patterns (e.g. daily, weekly, annual cycles), a stable social order and a consistency of physical places that an individual might inhabit.

Kielhofner (2008) presented two components of habituation. These are habits and internalized roles. *Habits* are patterns of behaviour that have a level of consistency about them and are often performed automatically. That is, the decision to engage in them and, often, to carry them out requires little thought. In addition, once commenced, habits require low levels of conscious effort, which frees up thought for other things while undertaking habitual activity. Habits rely on a familiarity with the environment that allows people to internalize rules for behaviour. When these rules have not been developed, often because the environment (or aspects of it) is novel, people are unable to respond in habitual ways.

The advantage of habits is both the freeing up of conscious thought for other things and, often, efficiency of response. For example, where habits have developed from action that has been modified over time within the same

6

context, they can result in efficient and effective behavioural responses to that environment. Expertise in a particular area may be a result of this process, in that, experts often appear to know what to do and are able to act with little apparent thought (respond habitually). It is only when something about the situation presents itself as novel that experts seem to need to engage in problem solving and deciding the best course of action.

Kielhofner (2008) identified three types of habits. First, the term *habits of occupational performance* refers to how people habitually perform routine activities. People develop habitual ways of doing daily activities such as dressing and bathing, as well as other frequently performed activities such as cooking, eating, and working. Second, people develop *habits of routine*. This refers to how people use time and space and how these ways become routinized. These routines can apply to different periods of time. For example, they could be daily (or within the day), weekly such as routines related to activities such as work or school (i.e. when you are working/studying and when you are having time off), seasonal (e.g. farmers), annual and so forth. Third, people develop *habits of style*. This refers to one's typical way of being in the world. Some examples that Kielhofner gave were whether a person typically attended to details or preferred to look at the broader picture, and whether they were prompt or procrastinating, quiet or talkative and trusting or cautious.

Over the course of the lifespan, habits can remain relatively stable or change. For example, some habits are considered socially acceptable at certain ages but not others. For an individual, some habits might serve an adaptive purpose at some times or in some circumstances and might gain an unwanted response in other situations. Some habits are the result of socialization and others are more related to the individual's particular experiences and ways of living.

The second component of habituation is *internalized roles*. The social system surrounding a person influences the roles that the person might desire, choose, be expected to fulfil or be prevented from obtaining. Roles powerfully influence the way human occupation is performed. As Kielhofner (2008) suggested, the process of internalizing roles "means taking on an identity, an outlook, and actions that belong to that role. Consequently, an internalized role is the incorporation of a socially and/or personally defined status and a related cluster of attitudes and actions" (p. 59).

In MOHO, an important aspect of internalized roles is role identification. Roles contribute to a person's self-identity. As Kielhofner (2008) stated, "identifying with any role means internalizing both what attributes society assigns to the role and one's personal interpretation of that role" (p. 60). When people take on roles they gain feedback about both their own perceptions of how well they have fulfilled those roles and the perceptions of others in society. All of this feedback contributes to how people think and feel about themselves. Internalized roles also provide people with "an internalised script" (Kielhofner, 2008, p. 60) that guides their behaviour by providing an understanding of the expectations of others and of themselves.

Kielhofner (2008) also proposed that roles organize occupations by: (1) influencing the style and content of people's actions; (2) shaping what people do; and (3) giving organization to time and space (e.g. by being in a certain role at a certain time in a certain place). Roles change over time, as people grow and mature, change their interests and plans, and as the context in which they live changes or their abilities change. As roles change, people's occupational engagement and performance will also change. An individual's capacity for performance and his or her experience of performance contribute to his or her ability to carry out roles and are described in the following section.

## PERFORMANCE CAPACITY AND THE LIVED BODY

In this third component of MOHO, the focus moves from the volition to act and the habits and roles that support and surround action to the action itself. In MOHO, action, referred to as performance, is discussed in terms of the capacity for performance and the embodied experience of performance. The phenomenological term "the lived body" is used to label this embodied experience.

Performance capacity refers to "the ability to do things" (Kielhofner, 2008, p. 68) and is conceptualized as having objective and subjective components. *Objective components* of performance capacity include the capacities of body systems such as musculoskeletal, neurological and cardiopulmonary systems, amongst others, as well as cognitive abilities. Kielhofner (2008) identified that other occupational therapy conceptual practice models detail performance capacities in greater depth by providing "specific explanations of physical and mental components and their contribution to performance" (p. 18). Examples include motor control models, cognitive approaches, etc. In contrast, MOHO provides little detail about these objective performance components, but emphasizes that performance capacity has both objective and subjective aspects.

*Subjective experience* refers to how the individual experiences performance and is understood to shape that experience. Kielhofner (2008) viewed attention to subjective experience as a neglected aspect of performance in occupational therapy, claiming that "focusing on the subjective aspect of performance capacity is complementary to the traditional objective approach" (p. 69). He referred to objective approaches as viewing performance capacity "from the outside" and subjective experience of performance capacity as viewed from the "inside" (p. 69). However, he proposed that, when occupational therapists ask people about their subjective experiences, they are actually doing so in order to build "an objective picture of performance capacity" (p. 69).

In the fourth edition of MOHO, the concept of subjective aspects of performance capacity is mainly discussed in contrast to objective performance components without providing much detail about what subjective aspects of performance includes. Therefore, it is unclear whether the subjective experience of performance capacity is conceptualized as separate to or a part of the other concept related to this component of human occupation, "the lived body".

The term *lived body* comes from phenomenology (a discipline of philosophy) and refers to the body *as it is lived* or experienced. It has been used in occupational therapy to refer to the embodied experience of performance (Mattingly & Fleming, 1994), that is, the fact that we live and move in a particular body, which shapes our experience of action. Subjective performance components might be conceptualized as part of the lived body. In explaining

Model of human occupation

the concept of the lived body, Kielhofner (2008) made reference to the philosopher Merleau-Ponty: "unlike the objective approach which describes performance from a detached, objective perspective, he [Merleau-Ponty] emphasized a phenomenological approach that considered subjective experience as fundamental to understanding human perception, cognition, and action" (p. 70).

"The lived body" emphasizes that the body is the vehicle through which life is lived and performance is experienced. Therefore, the capacity for and carrying out of performance is dependent on each individual's particular body. Phenomenology emphasizes that, in ordinary experience, the body forms the invisible background against which people attend to the occupations they are performing. The focus of attention is on the occupation rather than the body's participation in it. When people acquire impairments or have changes to their capacities, the body often comes to the foreground and can become the focus of attention.

In explaining the implications of the lived body for understanding human occupation, Kielhofner (2008) stated, "the lived body concept underscores two fundamental ideas" (p. 70). These are that (1) from the lived body perspective, there is a unity of mind and body (in that we experience our body and mind in an integrated way, as part of our bodies) and that (2) subjective experience of performance is fundamental to performance (we experience our own action as a part of *us* rather than as something objective and separate). Kielhofner argued that insufficient attention has been paid in occupational therapy to the lived experience of human occupation compared to its objective components.

## ENVIRONMENT

In MOHO, the term environment refers to "the particular physical and social, cultural, economic, and political features of one's contexts that impact upon the motivation, organisation, and performance of occupation" (Kielhofner, 2008, p. 86). As this definition emphasizes, the context within which an individual performs occupation shapes all three components of human performance – volition, habituation and performance – which motivate, organize and carry out occupation, respectively. Environments can provide opportunities and resources for occupation whilst also placing demands and constraints on it. In these ways, it is an important factor in shaping performance of occupation. Kielhofner referred to this process as "environmental impact" (p. 88).

Kielhofner (2008) presented a view of occupation in which a person is surrounded by four factors – spaces, objects, occupational forms or tasks, and social groups. Encompassing all of these are culture and its economic and political conditions. The person and the four factors surrounding the person are understood to be mutually influencing and the three conditions of the broader context influence all of the other factors.

*Spaces* refer to the physical contexts that shape behaviour. They have unique properties that influence what is done within them. These spaces could be man-made or part of the natural environment. *Objects* are "naturally occurring or fabricated things with which people interact and whose properties influence what they do with them" (Kielhofner, 2008, p. 88). Different types of objects lend themselves to different types of manipulation. For example, raw materials might tend to encourage imaginative play in children, whereas other objects are designed for specific purposes and are likely to shape their use accordingly. *Occupational forms and tasks* is a reference to Nelson's (1988) distinction between the things people do and the doing of them, which he called occupational form and performance, respectively. As Kielhofner (2008) stated, "the notion of form refers to the specific manner, actions, meanings, and so on that characterize doing something. When we perform, we go through or enact the form" (p. 92). He defined occupational forms/tasks as "conventionalised sequences of action that are at once coherent, oriented to a purpose, sustained in collective knowledge, culturally recognizable, and named" (p. 93). In discussing this definition he emphasized that occupational forms become conventionalized because there is usually a typical way to do them within a particular culture. *Social groups* provide the context within which much action occurs. They are influential in that they shape people's values, beliefs, interests and behaviours. The interactions in which people engage can be formal and informal, may be as small as a dyad and can influence what each person does.

Surrounding and influencing the person and all four factors in the environment is the broader cultural context with its economic and political conditions. Kielhofner (2008) described culture as "a pervasive feature of the environment" (p. 95) in which beliefs, values, norms, customs and so forth are shared and passed on through generations. Societies have cultural and sub cultural values and individuals will internalize these values to different extents. As part of the ways that societies are organized, economic and political factors influence what people do through the opportunities and resources people have (or do not have) access to and the demands and expectations that are placed on them according to their position within the society.

## DIMENSIONS OF DOING

All of these factors, both those internal to the person – volition, habituation and performance capacity – and the environment in which people live, influence what people do and how they do it. MOHO identified three dimensions of doing, all of which are influenced by volition, habituation, personal capacity and environmental conditions (context). These are occupational participation, occupational performance and skill. First, *occupational participation* refers to "engaging in work, play, or activities of daily living that are part of one's socio-cultural context and that are desired and/or necessary to one's well-being" (Kielhofner, 2008, p. 101). Occupational participation refers to broad categories of doing, includes both performance and its subjective experience and has both personal and social significance. Kielhofner (2008) emphasized that the way participation is understood in MOHO is consistent with how it is used in the International Classification of Functioning, Disability and Health (ICF) and the Occupational Therapy Practice Framework (OTPF). The second dimension of doing is *occupational performance*. Using Nelson's concepts of occupational form and performance, Kielhofner described occupational performance as "literally going through the form" (p. 103) of occupation, that is, doing an occupation. Third, the *skill* dimension refers to those skills that are required to perform the occupation. In MOHO these are categorized as motor skills (related to moving self or objects), process skills (logically sequencing actions over time) and communication and interaction skills (conveying needs and intentions and acting with others). As mentioned, volition, habituation, performance capacity and context impact upon all three dimensions of doing.

## LIFESPAN PERSPECTIVE

MOHO also emphasizes that human occupation changes over time as age and circumstances change and that it needs to be understood from a whole-of-life perspective. Drawing upon narrative theory, Kielhofner et al. (2008) commented that, "people conduct and draw meaning from life by locating themselves in unfolding narratives that integrate their past, present, and future selves" (p. 110). Lives have a temporal dimension and people have a biographical history that shapes their interpretations and behaviours in the present. They also think, feel and act in the present according to their goals and aspirations for the future.

Kielhofner et al. (2008) presented plot and metaphor as elements of narrative that people use to integrate their lives as a whole and create meaning. *Plot* gives narrative its structure and provides the temporal linking of events into an integrated whole. The authors gave examples of different plots that might characterize a person's life narrative, such as tragic plots (with a steep downward turn) and melodramatic plots (with a series of ups and downs). They provided three examples of the overall shape of a narrative, progressive (upward), regressive (downward) and stable (slight ups and downs around a middle point), that will influence a person's interpretation of individual events. For example, if people's life narratives are generally progressive or stable, they are more likely to interpret a particular event positively than someone with a regressive shape to their life narrative.

*Metaphor* is a figure of speech in which something familiar is used to substitute for something else. They are useful for conveying a depth of meaning that would be difficult to express using description alone. Often metaphors carry meanings that relate to the broader culture or society, so they are often imbued with shared meanings. Kielhofner et al. (2008) proposed that metaphors can be useful in making sense of difficulties and challenges and stated, "in pinpointing the essential nature of life's problems, struggles, and dilemmas, they also imply how they can be solved or overcome" (p. 112).

Using the concept of a narrative organization of life, Kielhofner et al. (2008) used the term *occupational narrative* to refer to "a story (both told and enacted) that integrates across time one's unfolding volition, habituation, performance capacity, and environments through plots and metaphors that sum up and assign meaning to these elements" (p. 113). Occupational narratives would be one part of a person's life narrative that relates to what they do and how this impacts upon their occupational identity and sense of occupational competence.

The concept of occupational narrative emphasizes the temporal nature of human occupation. MOHO presents human occupation as a complex phenomenon with a range of dimensions. It results from the complex interaction between unique individuals – with their own particular motivations, interests and values (volition); habits, routines and internalized roles (habituation);

and capabilities and experiences of themselves and their lives (performance capacity and the lived experience) – and their environments over time. These interactions can be relatively stable or marked by upward or downward trends over time.

The structure of MOHO differs greatly from many of the other occupational therapy models. It deals with the interaction between a person and his or her context when doing things. Like most occupational therapy models, it emphasizes the various ways that the context in which occupation is performed shapes that performance. However, the detailed analysis of volition and habituation, attention to the narrative aspects of occupational life and the relative lack of detail about performance sets it apart from many of the other occupational therapy models of practice. The section that follows discusses the historical development of the model, particularly in relation to its theoretical foundations.

## HISTORICAL DESCRIPTION OF MODEL'S DEVELOPMENT

MOHO is an occupational therapy model that has had a very long publication history. According to Kielhofner (2008), MOHO was first published in 1980 in a series of four articles in the *American Journal of Occupational Therapy*. He described the model as "the product of three occupational therapy practitioners attempting to articulate concepts that guided their practice" (Kielhofner, 2008, p. 1). As a single volume, MOHO has been published in four editions, commencing in 1985 and spanning the intervening decades to 2008. It is a conceptual model that has influenced occupational therapy theory and practice over, possibly, the most sustained period of the profession's history.

The Model of Human Occupation is an important model in occupational therapy because it was developed at a time when occupational therapy was very influenced by the ideas of the biomedical model of health. According to Madigan and Parent (1985), Mary Reilly, from the University of Southern California (USC), had been cautioning occupational therapy since the late 1950s that its alignment with medicine was too narrowing. Reilly's argument had been that medicine's focus was on the prevention and reduction of disease and illness, whereas occupational therapy dealt with the process of helping people to adapt their lives to develop and preserve life satisfaction "through work and social development" (Madigan & Parent, 1985, p. vii). Reilly's theory of occupational behaviour guided research and teaching at USC for a number of decades and was an important influence in the development of MOHO.

In 1985, Madigan and Parent explained that the MOHO publication was "the latest compilation of many persons' efforts to build and apply a theory unique to occupational therapy" (Madigan & Parent, 1985, p. vii). At that time, Kielhofner explained the need for a model by saying that the extensive development that occurred in the occupational behaviour tradition led to the development of many concepts. He stated, "Since the number of concepts grew to be large and somewhat cumbersome, it became necessary to develop models of practice which integrated these concepts into a workable format. The model of human occupation began as one such model which sought to build upon the existing occupational behaviour tradition" (Kielhofner, cited in Madigan & Parent, 1985, p. xviii).

It appears that, at the time of the 1985 publication, it was unclear whether Kielhofner's MOHO was "an extension and further evolution of occupational behaviour theory" or whether it was a new direction in theory (Madigan & Parent, 1985, p. ix). While it was clear that the model flowed logically from occupational behaviour in terms of its major concepts of "role, interests, values, personal causation, intrinsic motivation, and environment, to name a few" (Madigan & Parent, 1985, p. ix), Reed was also cited as taking the position that MOHO was different from occupational behaviour theory (although clearly developed from it). Over time, as the model has been further developed, its difference from occupational behaviour theory has been demonstrated clearly.

In some ways, the model has changed enormously over time while its overall structure has remained similar. A major change has been the way its basis in systems theory has been described over time. A discussion of the particular aspects of systems theory that influenced the model in its first edition will make evident how the model came to be structured as it is, with the components of volition, habituation and performance capacity. Volition, habituation and performance were originally described as subsystems in 1985 and conceptualized as having a hierarchical relationship. However, in the second edition they are described as a heterarchy of subcomponents (explained later) and in the fourth edition (2008) they are called "interrelated components" (p. 12) and are conceptualized as non-hierarchical and mutually influencing.

In explaining the systems basis to the model, in all four editions Kielhofner contrasted it with a mechanistic perspective. In the third edition, Kielhofner (2002) explained that the model had originally been developed in response to the profession's previous alignment with medicine, with its mechanistic understanding of health. (As explained in the introduction to this book, the adoption of systems theory in the area of health allowed for a broader understanding in Western countries of the factors that affect an individual's health.)

The first two editions of MOHO explained various aspects of systems theory as the basis for its understanding of human occupation. In the first edition, the model was presented as based on open systems theory. In this edition, Kielhofner (1985) contrasted open and closed systems theory by showing that closed systems (e.g. machines) wear down with use (entropy) while open systems have the capacity to build up and become more complex (negative entropy). The implication in terms of occupation is that humans can develop and become more complex through doing.

The second edition of MOHO is based on dynamic systems theory. In the first edition, volition, habituation and performance were conceptualized as subsystems and understood to have a hierarchical relationship where the higher systems command the lower systems and the lower systems constrain the higher systems. Thus, for example, volition was considered the highest subsystem and thought to command, but be constrained by, the lower ones.

A major difference between dynamic and open systems theory is that, in dynamic systems, the organism is considered to have the capacity to reorganize itself. The way systems maintain themselves in optimal conditions is referred to as their "steady state" (Kielhofner 1985, p. 7). In an open systems view, systems maintain their structure. However, dynamic systems theory assumes that organisms are able to reorganize themselves and become more complex. Prigogine and Stengers (1984), in their book *Order out of Chaos*, used the example of water flowing in a stream to illustrate the assumption of the capacity to reorganize in dynamic systems theory. As water flows over rocks, it becomes increasingly destabilized and chaotic (splashes, etc.). However, as its steady state becomes more and more disturbed, it can reorganize itself, for example, into a whirlpool, which is organized differently from the currents in the original stream.

Consistent with this change from open systems theory to dynamic systems theory, the relationship between the subsystems of MOHO (volition, habituation and performance) in the second edition were no longer considered to be a hierarchy but a heterarchy. As Kielhofner (1995) explained, "The concept of heterarchy recognizes that systems arrange themselves according to the demands of situations in which they are performing, not according to a pre-ordained or fixed structure" (p. 34).

The concept of heterarchy was applied to MOHO through the assumption of "dynamical assembly of behaviour" (Kielhofner, 1995, p. 14). When using a mechanistic metaphor (common in biomedicine) the assumption is that structure causes function. This suggests that behaviour can be predicted according to the structure of the organism. However, when applied to humans, structure is unable to explain their *potential* for behaviour and how humans select from all of these possible behaviours. As Kielhofner (1995) stated, "Humans perform in an almost infinite variety of emotional, cognitive, and physical circumstances" (p. 15) and he proposed that no two instances of performing the same activity are exactly the same because humans are able to assemble their behaviour differently as the circumstances demand. Just as the water flowing across rocks can reorganize itself to suit the surroundings, so too humans engage in "self-organisation" through occupation. As Kielhofner (1995) stated, "When we work, play, and perform the tasks of daily life, we are not merely engaging in occupational behaviour, we are organising ourselves. We use our bodies and minds in the contexts of occupations, organizing them accordingly. We create our motor abilities, our self-concepts, social identities in our occupations. Occupational behaviour is self-making." (p. 22.)

The model's basis in systems theory was discussed most overtly and in most detail in the first two editions. In the third and fourth editions, a systems perspective (as a general concept) is mentioned (rather than explained in detail) and is mainly contrasted with a mechanistic perspective (the main purpose appears to be distinguishing MOHO from the reductionist perspective of biomedicine). Three concepts of systems theory are emphasized in both later editions. These are heterarchy, emergence and control parameter.

First, *heterarchy* can be contrasted with hierarchy. As explained before, hierarchy refers to an organizational structure in which the higher levels command the lower levels and the lower levels constrain the higher levels. In contrast, heterarchy assumes a non-hierarchical organization in which the components function according to the needs of the whole. That is, components contribute to the whole according to their capacities and the relationship between different components is reorganized according to the requirements of the whole. In relation to MOHO, this means that the four components – volition, habituation, performance and environment – are assembled (or called upon) according to the occupational requirements in the situation. Second, Kielhofner (2008) defined *emergence* as "the principle that complex actions, thoughts, and feelings spontaneously arise out of the interactions of several components" (p. 25). This suggests that these actions, thoughts and feelings are not predetermined but *emerge* from the combination of volition, habituation, performance and environment (which will be uniquely assembled for each situation). Third, a *control parameter* is a factor that changes the whole dynamic when it changes. Kielhofner described it as a "critical change" that results in a "different emergent behaviour" (p. 26). What this means is that a change in any of volition, habituation, performance and/or the environment will result in the need for a different behavioural response.

The second way that MOHO has developed over its four editions relates to performance. In the first edition, performance was considered the lowest level in the hierarchy of subcomponents within the person. Therefore, it was initially conceptualized as commanded by volition and habituation and able to constrain both. In later editions, the performance component became labelled *performance capacity and the lived experience*. This relabelling shows a shift in attention to the capacity to perform and an emphasis on subjective experience of performance, both of which centre on the process of and potential for performing rather than just performance as an outcome. In including the concept of the lived experience, the MOHO developers appear to have been influenced by the work of Cheryl Mattingly, an anthropologist who introduced this concept to occupational therapy during her work on the AOTA clinical reasoning project in the 1980s (see Mattingly & Fleming, 1994). Mattingly discussed the concept of the lived experience when describing the work of the French philosopher Merleau-Ponty on phenomenology and embodied experience. Phenomenology distinguishes between an event and a person's *experience* of that event and Merleau-Ponty further emphasized that a person experiences the world *through* his or her body. Thus, the capacity to perform and the individual's experience of that capacity and of performing are important aspects of the later editions of MOHO.

The third major way that MOHO has progressed over time is through the development of its tools to assist practice. While only a brief overview is provided here, readers are encouraged to refer to the fourth edition, which provides a variety of chapters discussing the occupational therapy process, assessment and intervention. First, Kielhofner and Forsyth (2008a) presented a six-step therapeutic reasoning process. This consisted of: (1) generating questions to guide information gathering; (2) gathering information on or with the client; (3) creating a conceptualization of the client that includes strengths and challenges; (4) identifying goals and plans for client engagement and therapeutic strategies; (5) implementing and reviewing therapy; and (6) collecting information to assess outcomes. Second, a variety of assessment tools have been developed to assist with the collecting of information about the important concepts within MOHO. Table 6.1 provides a list of assessment tools and the MOHO concepts they address. Assessments use the methods of observation, self-report and interview to collect information.

Table 6.1 MOHO assessments (adapted from Kielhofner 2008, pp. 160–161)

| Concepts addressed by the assessment | Occupational adaptation | | Volition | | | Habituation | | Skills | | | Performance | Partici- pation | Environment | |
|---|---|---|---|---|---|---|---|---|---|---|---|---|---|---|
| Assessment | Identity | Competence | Personal causation | Values | Interests | Roles | Habits | Motor | Process | Communi- cation/ Interaction | | | Physical | Social |
| Assessment of communication & interaction skills | | | | | | | | | | x | | | | |
| Assessment of motor & process skills | | | | | | | | x | x | | | | | |
| Assessment of occupational functioning | | | x | x | x | x | x | x | x | x | | | | |
| Child occupational self-assessment | | x | x | x | x | x | x | x | x | x | x | x | | |
| Interest checklist | | | | | x | | | | | | | | | |
| Model of Human Occupation screening tool | | | x | x | x | x | x | x | x | x | x | x | x | x |

(Continued)

**Table 6.1**  *MOHO assessments (adapted from Kielhofner 2008, pp. 160–161)—Cont'd*

| Concepts addressed by the assessment | Occupational adaptation | | Volition | | | Habituation | | Skills | | | Performance | Partici-pation | Environment | |
|---|---|---|---|---|---|---|---|---|---|---|---|---|---|---|
| Assessment | Identity | Competence | Personal causation | Values | Interests | Roles | Habits | Motor | Process | Communication/ Interaction | Performance | Participation | Physical | Social |
| NIH activity record | | | × | × | × | × | × | | | | × | × | | |
| Occupational circumstances assessment – interview & rating scale | | | × | × | × | × | × | | | | × | × | × | × |
| Occupational performance history interview II | × | × | × | × | × | × | × | | | | | × | | |
| Occupational questionnaire | | | × | × | × | × | × | | | | | × | | |
| Occupational self-assessment | | × | × | × | × | × | × | × | × | × | × | × | × | × |
| Occupational therapy psychosocial assessment of learning | | | × | × | × | × | × | | | | × | × | × | × |

| Assessment | | | | | | | | | |
|---|---|---|---|---|---|---|---|---|---|
| Paediatric interest profile | × | × | × | | | | | | × |
| Paediatric volitional questionnaire | × | × | × | | | | × | × | × |
| Role checklist | | × | × | | | | | | |
| School setting interview | | | | × | | × | × | × | × |
| Short child occupational profile | × | × | × | × | × | × | × | × | × |
| Volitional questionnaire | × | × | × | | | | | | |
| Worker role interview | × | × | × | × | | | × | × | × |
| Work environment impact scale | | | | | | | × | × | × |

Third, regarding intervention, Kielhofner and Forsyth (2008b) provided nine types of client effort that could contribute to change in occupational engagement. They proposed that it is important for occupational therapists to consider these when working with clients. These are:

- Choice and decision-making are important aspects of clients' engagement in occupation
- Clients need to commit to engage in the necessary action for the time that is required to make a change
- Clients need to be prepared to explore options for occupation, and their feelings and experiences related to them
- Clients need to locate "novel information, alternatives for action, new attitudes, and new feelings that provide solutions for and/or give meaning to occupational performance and participation" (p. 173)
- Clients need to have the opportunity to negotiate about therapy
- Clients may be more successful in meeting their goals for occupational engagement if they plan how they will approach this goal
- Occupational change requires practice
- Clients often have to engage in re-examination of "perception, feelings, beliefs, and patterns of acting that are no longer valid or that have led to difficulties" (p. 177)
- Clients often have to sustain effort over time and despite difficulties and uncertainty

Kielhofner and Forsyth (2008c) also identified nine therapeutic strategies for enabling change. These were:

- Validating clients' experiences, perspectives and efforts
- Identifying factors that could facilitate change
- Giving feedback
- Providing advice
- Negotiating with clients
- Structuring clients' occupational engagement
- Coaching, which includes instructing, demonstrating, guiding, and providing verbal and/or physical prompts
- Encouraging clients to explore, practise and persist in their efforts
- Providing physical support

They proposed that these therapeutic strategies are used to influence occupational engagement and to complement the different types of effort that clients can contribute to the therapeutic encounter. They also emphasized that the strategies identified are based on MOHO theory, so occupational therapists using MOHO should be familiar with its theory.

In summary, MOHO has changed and developed over three decades. While some concepts have remained from the original edition (volition, habituation and performance), the theoretical assumptions about humans and their occupation have changed over that time. That is, humans were conceptualized initially as open systems, then as dynamic systems and then as having inter-related components. Over time, the model has increasingly emphasized the capacity for people to organize their component skills uniquely as the occupation and context requires.

See Box 6.1.

> ### BOX 6.1  MOHO memory aid
>
> Occupational identity: As an occupational being, what is this person's sense of who he/she is, has been and will/wants to be in the future?
>
> Occupational competence: How well has this person maintained a pattern of occupational engagement and participation that is consistent with his/her sense of occupational identity?
>
> Participation: In what ways does this person participate (or want to participate) in his/her sociocultural context through work, play and activities of daily living in response to his/her needs/wants and society's expectations?
>
> Performance: What occupational forms/tasks is this person able/unable to do in the areas of work, play and activities of daily living?
>
> Skills: How well does this person's motor, process and/or communication/interaction skills match what he/she wants/needs to do?
>
> Volition: What are this person's motivations, values and interests? To what degree does he/she feel able to influence his/her occupations, circumstances and environment?
>
> Habituation: What roles does the person need/want to fulfil? How well do this person's habits support his/her ability to engage in occupations and roles in his/her particular environment?
>
> Performance capacity: How do this person's body systems support performance? How does he/she experience engagement in occupation? What is this person's embodied experience of acting in the world?
>
> Environment: How does the environment impact on this person's occupational engagement (opportunities and resources that it provides, demands and constraints that it imposes)?
>
> Adapted from Kielhofner, 2008, p. 148.

## CONCLUSION

MOHO is the occupational therapy model of practice that has the longest continuous progress, with it being updated and developed for three decades to date. It was first created to provide organization to many of the concepts associated with the occupational behaviour tradition. The first two editions situated its conceptual basis within systems theory and focused on the person as comprised of subsystems that influenced performance. These subsystems were volition, habituation and performance. At the time of its early development, it was one of the few models of practice that attended to the motivational aspects of human occupation. Therefore, it was quite influential in contributing to an understanding of people's occupation that went beyond a focus on the body and impairments to sensorimotor, cognitive and psychosocial functions.

The third and fourth editions of MOHO de-emphasized systems theory as a theoretical basis, and focused increasingly on the relationship between the person and the environment during occupation. While the concepts of volition, habituation and performance remained, they were no longer conceptualized as components of a system. Instead, they were used to understand how people "select, organise and undertake their occupations" (Kielhofner, 2008, p. 12). In these two editions, these three concepts were considered, along with the environment, as part of a set of four major concepts used to understand human occupation. These four concepts were also combined with participation, performance, skill, occupational identity, occupational competence and occupational adaptation in the later two editions.

A unique feature of MOHO is the substantial development of assessment tools that has taken place over time. No other model of practice has developed these types of tools to this extent. Consistent with the model's focus on subjective experience, these assessments use observation, self-report and interview. The model also outlines processes to guide intervention.

## MAJOR WORKS

Kielhofner, G. (Ed.), 1985. A model of human occupation: Theory and application. Williams & Wilkins, Baltimore, MD.

Kielhofner, G., 1995. A model of human occupation: Theory and application, second ed. Williams & Wilkins, Baltimore, MD.

Kielhofner, G., 2002. A model of human occupation: Theory and application, third ed. Lippincott Williams & Wilkins, Baltimore, MD.

Kielhofner, G., 2008. A model of human occupation: Theory and application, fourth ed. Lippincott Williams & Wilkins, Baltimore, MD.

## REFERENCES

Csikszentmihalyi, M., 1990. Flow: The psychology of optimal experience. Harper & Rowe, New York.

Kielhofner, G. (Ed.), 1985. A model of human occupation: Theory and application. Williams & Wilkins, Baltimore, MD.

Kielhofner, G., 1995. A model of human occupation: Theory and application, second ed. Williams & Wilkins, Baltimore, MD.

Kielhofner, G., 2002. A model of human occupation: Theory and application, third ed. Lippincott Williams & Wilkins, Baltimore, MD.

Kielhofner, G., 2008. A model of human occupation: Theory and application, fourth ed. Lippincott Williams & Wilkins, Baltimore, MD.

Kielhofner, G., Forsyth, K., 2008a. Therapeutic reasoning: planning, implementing, and evaluating the outcomes of therapy. In: Kielhofner, G. (Ed.), A model of human occupation: Theory and application, fourth ed. Lippincott Williams & Wilkins, Baltimore, MD, pp. 143–154.

Kielhofner, G., Forsyth, K., 2008b. Occupational engagement: How clients achieve change. In: Kielhofner, G. (Ed.), A model of human occupation: Theory and application, fourth ed. Lippincott Williams & Wilkins, Baltimore, MD, pp. 171–184.

Kielhofner, G., Forsyth, K., 2008c. Therapeutic strategies for enabling change. In: Kielhofner G. (Ed.), A model of human occupation: Theory and application, fourth ed. Lippincott Williams & Wilkins, Baltimore, MD, pp. 185–203.

Kielhofner, G., Borell, L., Holzmuller, R., et al., 2008. Crafting occupational life. In: Kielhofner, G. (Ed.), A model of human occupation: Theory and application, fourth ed. Lippincott Williams & Wilkins, Baltimore, MD, pp. 110–125.

Madigan, M.J., Parent, L.H., 1985. Preface. In: Kielhofner, G. (Ed.), A model of human occupation: Theory and application. Williams & Wilkins, Baltimore, MD.

Mattingly, C., Fleming, M.H., 1994. Clinical reasoning: forms of inquiry in a therapeutic practice. F.A. Davis, Philadelphia, PA.

Nelson, D., 1988. Occupation: Form and performance. Am. J. Occup. Ther. 42 (10), 633–641.

Prigogine, I., Stengers, I., 1984. Order out of chaos: Man's new dialogue with nature. New Science Library, Boulder, CO.

# Kawa model

7

The Kawa (River in Japanese) model was developed by Michael Iwama, a Japanese-Canadian occupational therapist and social scientist, in conjunction with a group of Japanese occupational therapists. The Kawa model is the most recently developed of those models reviewed in this book (although some models have since been updated). The Kawa model was presented at various conferences in the early 2000s and the main text outlining the model was published in 2006. The model was originally developed in response to a perceived need for an occupational therapy model that was appropriate and useful in Japanese occupational therapy practice contexts. Therefore, the challenge for Western readers when learning about this model is to understand it in the context of the culture within and for which it was developed. The Kawa model uses the metaphor of a river with various elements such as water, rock, driftwood and the river floor and river walls. The potential trap for many readers is to take this metaphor and its elements, and view them from an individualist perspective. Understood in this way, the model could look like any other occupational therapy model that deals with the person, environment and occupation. However, by understanding the assumptions about the nature of self and agency that are embedded within collectivist cultures such

**159**

© 2011 Elsevier Ltd.
DOI: 10.1016/B978-0-7234-3494-8.00007-3

as Japanese and various indigenous societies, Western readers are better able to understand the significance of the various elements of this model. To facilitate this process, comments are made throughout the description of the model that emphasize a culturally appropriate understanding of each phenomenon. Reference is also made to the distinction Iwama made between *collectivist* and *existential* perspectives. The former is the perspective characterized by many East Asian and indigenous cultures. The latter characterizes the individualist approach common in Western cultures.

## MAIN CONCEPTS AND DEFINITIONS OF TERMS

The Kawa model is structured around the metaphor of a river and its elements. It uses the image of the water flowing through a river to represent 'life energy' or 'life flow'. In this model, the purpose of occupational therapy is to facilitate this life flow in the context of a harmonious balance with all aspects of the river. The river itself is used to describe a person's life history (Figure 7.1) and cross-sections of the river at different times in the person's history (Figures 7.2 and 7.3) can reveal the elements in the river. These elements are the river floor and walls, rocks, driftwood and the spaces between these. Each element represents an aspect of the person's life circumstances. The water flows through the channels that are created by the relative positions and sizes of the other elements. Change can occur in the river by alteration of the position, size and shape of the elements to increase or decrease the flow of the water. This potential for change is the basis for occupational therapy intervention.

The river is used to represent the flow or energy of life. It could refer to the life of an individual person, a family or the life of an organization (Iwama,

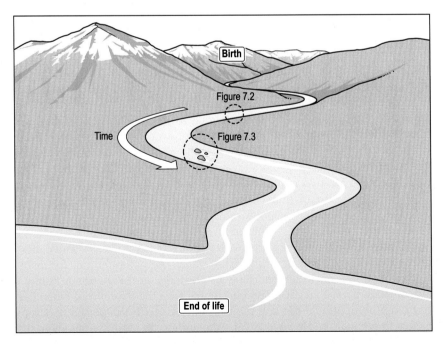

**FIG 7.1** The river. *From Iwama, The Kawa Model (2006) Churchill Livingstone, with permission from Elsevier Ltd.*

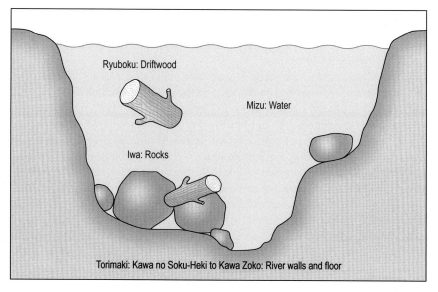

**FIG 7.2** Elements of the river. *From Iwama, The Kawa Model (2006) Churchill Livingstone, with permission from Elsevier Ltd.*

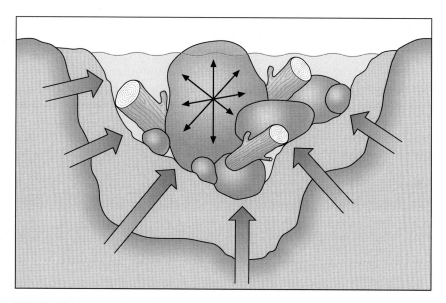

**FIG 7.3** Elements constricting water flow. *From Iwama, The Kawa Model (2006) Churchill Livingstone, with permission from Elsevier Ltd.*

2006). In the metaphor of a river, the importance of context in shaping the river is emphasized. Rivers start because the moisture from rain and melting snow etcetera flows toward the lowest point of the land. Depending on the surrounding geography, rivers commence with varying amounts and types of water flow. They also flow towards lakes (some of which might be dry in lands such as Australia) and the sea. The course that the river takes depends on the unique combination of the surrounding geography, the strength of the river's water flow and anything that lies in the river such as rocks and drift-wood. Similarly, the flow of the water can vary in different parts of the river as variations occur in the unique combination of the quality of the water flow and other elements of the river.

In the Kawa model, the river is used as a metaphor for the life journey, with birth being represented by the start of the river and end of life being the point at which the river flows into a larger body of water such as the sea. As Iwama (2006) explained, "An optimal state of well-being in one's life or *river*, can be metaphorically portrayed by an image of strong, deep, unimpeded flow" (p. 143). As a metaphor for life, the river shows that people's lives are shaped by the unique contexts into which they are born and live as well as aspects of their own character and skill. Just as the river makes twists and turns, people's lives change in a variety of ways. Some of these changes can be anticipated, some are unexpected, some are shaped by the surrounding con-text and others are primarily shaped by the flow of the water, which changes the shape of the river floor and walls. Sometimes the flow of people's lives is impeded by obstacles and at other times everything seems to flow easily. Some people are born into or live in circumstances that flow easily like a wide river and others' lives are characterized by obstacles that impact substantially upon their life flow.

While the river as a whole represents a person's life, a cross-section taken at various points of the river would show different arrangements of the ele-ments of the river. In certain places, the river might be wide and deep and the water flow might be largely unimpeded by obstacles. In other places, it might be narrow and flow over rocks or drop in waterfalls. And still other places, the water flow might become impeded by debris or rock barriers that make the water stagnant. Similarly, the same section of river will look different at different times if the rainfall has varied and the river might run strongly or be almost dried up. In the Kawa model, attention is paid to both the river as a whole and to cross-sections at different places. In the cross-sectional view, the various elements of the river are used as metaphors for different aspects of life.

## ELEMENTS OF THE RIVER

The first element in the Kawa model is the *water*. The element of the river used in the Kawa model to represent life energy or life flow is water, or *mizu* in Japanese. In many different cultures, water has symbolic meanings that relate to life. It is possible that water is a seemingly universal symbol of life because it is biologically essential for sustaining human life. Iwama (2006) highlighted that, while water is considered to be pure, cleansing and renewing and is often associated with the spirit, culturally specific meanings for water also abound throughout the world. He encouraged people to explore what water symbol-izes in the particular cultures with which they might be engaging.

Water has a fluidity that allows it to flow over, around and through a range of different obstacles and channels in its path. As a fluid, it has the capacity to both shape and be shaped by whatever surrounds or contains it. It can take on the shape of a container but it also has the power to shape things that it flows over or through. For example, the erosion that occurs in rocks that are exposed to water attests to its power to shape its surroundings. As Iwama (2006) stated, "Just as people's lives are bounded and shaped by their surroundings, people and circumstances, the water flowing as a river touches the rocks, walls and banks and all other elements of the river in a similar way to which the same elements affect the water's volume, shape and flow rate" (p. 144). He also explained how important this mutually influencing relationship between the water and its surroundings is to understanding collective culture. He stated, "collectively oriented people tend to place enormous value on the *self* embedded in relationships. There is greater value in 'belonging' and 'interdependence', than in unilateral agency and in individual determinism. In such experience, the interdependent self is deeply influenced and even determined by the surrounding social context, at a given time and place, in a similar way to which water in a river, at any given point, will vary in form, flow direction rate, volume and clarity." (p. 145.)

Water also has the capacity to fill the spaces between other things and only needs small spaces in which to flow. As a metaphor for life, this might suggest that life flow is possible in even the smallest of avenues. From the perspective of this metaphor, the task of an occupational therapist is to look at all aspects of the person's context of daily life and facilitate greater life flow. "When life energy or flow weakens, the occupational therapy client, whether defined as individual or collective, can be described as unwell, or in a state of disharmony" (Iwama, 2006, p. 144). An occupational therapist can use any elements of the river (and their combinations) to work towards facilitating life flow.

The next concepts are the *river walls and river floor*. In the Kawa model, the river walls and river floor are referred to as *kawa no soku-heki* and *kawa no zoko*, respectively. Just as the walls and floor of the river shape the course, depth and width of the river, these parts of the river are used in the Kawa model to refer to the contexts that surround clients, that is, their social and physical environments. Iwama (2006) made the point that "these are perhaps the most important determinants of a person's life flow in a collectivist social context because of the primacy afforded to the environmental context in determining the experiences of self and subsequent meanings of personal action" (p. 146).

In discussing the river walls and floor, Iwama mainly attended to the social environment, possibly because of the importance of emphasizing the nature of a collectivist society to a Western audience. He stressed that the social environment chiefly refers to those people with which clients have direct relationships and he gave examples of what the river walls and floor might represent, such as family members, pets (that are very important to them), friends, workmates, classmates and so forth. He also emphasized that, in some cultures, the memories of departed family members can exert an important influence on people and that, in some cases, conversing with such departed relatives might constitute an important occupation for particular clients.

When using the Kawa model, the various elements of the river have to be considered together for occupational therapists to gain the holist perspective for which they strive. Therefore, when thinking about the river walls and floor, it is important to understand that there is no particular shape that is 'optimal'. What matters is the amount of water that is able to flow through the combination, placement and interaction of the various elements of the river. For instance, rivers that have reasonably narrow or shallow walls and floor might allow for adequate water flow if there are no obstacles blocking its flow. Similarly, a deep river that has been dammed will restrict the river flow in a way that is unrelated to the natural shape of the walls and floor. Metaphorically, the environment will certainly shape the life flow of a person but this may be in a facilitatory or inhibitory way. Using the Kawa model, occupational therapists can look for ways to help shape the environment to facilitate the flow of the client's river and to enhance the harmony existing between clients and their contexts.

The third element of the Kawa model is *rocks*. The Japanese word *iwa*, which means large rocks or crags, is used in the Kawa model's representation of life circumstances that are perceived by the client to be problematic. These life circumstances are seen to impede life flow and are considered by the client to be difficult to remove. Just as rocks can disturb the flow of water because of their shape, size and placement in relation to the walls and floor of the river, rocks are used to represent such life circumstances in the lives of people. The rocks in a person's life might be challenges that derive from bodily impairments that, in a particular environment, impede their life energy. Using the river image metaphorically, the unique size and placement of this rock in relation to the shape of the river walls and floor might impede the flow of the water. However, in a river with differently shaped walls and floor, the same rock might have a minimal effect on the flow of the water. Thus, it is important when using the model to discuss with the client the extent to which potential obstacles to life flow are actually perceived as impacting upon his or her life.

Many of the examples of rocks provided in the major publication on the Kawa model (Iwama, 2006) relate to impairments of body structures and function such as low motivation, anxiety, depression and history of relapse – all symptoms and consequences of mental illness – and brachial nerve injury and pulmonary emphysema; while others relate to problems of performance such as difficulties with activities of daily living and self care. However, other rocks listed are money and human relations, which illustrate that obstacles in one's life can relate to things other than impairments of body structure and function. Each person's life circumstances and contexts of living are unique and will differ among people.

The fourth element of the river discussed in the Kawa model is *driftwood*. The image of driftwood, *ryuboku* in Japanese, is used to represent:

> personal attributes and resources, such as values (i.e. honesty, thrift), character
> (i.e. optimism, stubbornness), personality (i.e. reserved, outgoing), special skill
> (i.e. carpentry, public speaking), immaterial (i.e. friends, siblings) and material
> (i.e. wealth, special equipment) assets and living situation (rural and urban,
> shared accommodations, etc) that can positively or negatively affect the subject's
> circumstance and life flow. (Iwama, 2006, p. 149)

Some of these examples of *personal attributes and resources* refer to features of an individual while others relate to that individual's immediate context and circumstance. While driftwood is also described as representing personal assets and liabilities, the concept of personal attributes and resources probably conjures a better image of what the driftwood is used to represent in the model. The image of assets and liabilities is often interpreted from an existential perspective to refer to characteristics that are within the person rather than surrounding him or her whereas driftwood includes resources external to the person.

The utility of the concept of assets and liabilities lies in placing an emphasis on the fact that these attributes and resources can have a negative or positive effect on life flow. For example, Iwama (2006) provided a table listing examples of driftwood and, for each, positive and negative effects that each example might have on the life of an individual. Some of these are as follows: future expectations could have the positive effect of providing goals or something to look forward to, while potentially having negative effects by being a source of frustration, stress and worry; parents' advantaged financial status could have the positive effect of assisting with equipment purchases and required home renovations while also possibly facilitating increased dependency and contributing to a lack of skill development on the part of the client.

Compared with rocks, driftwood is considered to be less permanent and a more fluid situation within the river. Driftwood can be carried along with the water current and, depending on their shape and number, can become caught on the rocks or combine to create a dam that restricts the flow of the water. However, when carried by the strength of the water flow, they can also dislodge obstacles or carve channels in the river walls or floor, thereby increasing the flow of the water.

The final, but centrally important, element in the Kawa model is the *spaces* between obstructions. These are called *sukima* in Japanese and help us to understand the focus of occupational therapy from the perspective of this model. The elegant title of the section of book in which spaces is discussed is "*Sukima* (space between obstructions) where life energy still flows: The promise of occupational therapy" (p. 151). In the Kawa model, the concept of sukima is based on an understanding of occupational therapy as a strengths-based approach. Rather than focusing on the remediation of problems, sukima emphasizes the importance of understanding where life is flowing in a client's situation and strategically working to maximize that flow.

While reduction in the size and shape of obstacles might be a strategy that can be used to maximize the life flow, it becomes only one of many ways to enhance life flow in those places in the river where it already exists. Focusing on the spaces *between* objects rather than the objects themselves, the Kawa model emphasizes the potential to facilitate life flow in a range of ways including reducing the size and shape of problems, making channels in or changing the shape of the environment surrounding the client, and maximizing the power of the client's existing assets and resources. Using the metaphor of the river, the spaces where the water flows have the potential to increase through the friction that can wear away or dislodge those things that surround and impede its flow.

## THE RIVER METAPHOR

In explaining the relevance of the metaphor to occupational therapy practice, Iwama (2006) linked the concept of spaces to social roles and occupation. First he explained, by way of illustration, that a functional impairment such as arthritis might be represented in the model by a rock, and a social group or person might represent the river walls. The space between these two, through which the water flows, might represent a particular social role such as parent, worker or friend, etc. Second, he stated that, "the spaces through which life flows, is representative of 'occupation', from an Eastern perspective" (p. 151). This linking of social roles and occupation is useful in understanding an Eastern comprehension of occupation. In collectivist societies, human action takes its meaning from the person's position in society. Therefore, occupation becomes one vehicle through which individuals can fulfil their social roles. In other situations, for example, non-action might be the way that an individual can fulfil these roles.

Thinking about the river metaphor is useful in highlighting how the Kawa model is employed to understand a person's life flow and the role that occupational therapy might have in facilitating this. The society in which people live shapes the kinds of roles that a person has (i.e. shapes the form and direction of the river) and obstacles that might relate to the person and/or his or her circumstances (rocks) can impede the life flow of the person and his or her ability to fulfil those social roles. Aspects of the person's character, skills and circumstances (driftwood) are carried along by the water and may be able to flow through the river unimpeded or might become caught in the spaces between the river walls and floor and any rocks. Where driftwood contributes to a blockage of the river, it might impede the flow of water or its damming effect might combine with the force of the water to dislodge obstacles or divert the water flow through new channels in the river walls and floor.

The fact that the water is frequently able to find new channels through which to flow provides the "promise of occupational therapy" (Iwama, 2006, p. 151). It only takes a small space through which the water can flow to provide the potential for enhancing that life flow. Occupational therapists can use their creativity to work with the client or group and those that are connected to and are instrumental in shaping the client's social roles to seek ways of increasing the channels through which the water can flow. Using the Kawa model, occupational therapists are encouraged to view each cross-section of the river in a holistic way and keep in mind that the flow of water can be facilitated in a range of ways. Working to expand the current spaces through which water flows could be approached by exploring if there are any ways that the walls and floor of the river could be shaped to increase this space, whether rocks could be moved or reduced in size and how driftwood could best be used to enlarge the spaces that currently exist. The occupational therapist could also look for places where new channels of water could easily be opened up (e.g. new social roles that might be available). Thus, the river metaphor emphasizes that it is the unique combinations of and relations between the various elements of the river that form the basis for understanding a client's or group's current needs and the possibilities for addressing these needs within that particular life circumstance.

## HISTORICAL DESCRIPTION OF MODEL'S DEVELOPMENT

The Kawa model was originally developed by a group of Japanese occupational therapists as a model relevant to Japanese culture, characterized by collectivism and hierarchy. As occupational therapy is a profession that developed in Western countries, the Japanese occupational therapists found that many of the assumptions upon which the theoretical basis of the profession was founded differed from their own understanding of life and the nature of humans. Iwama (2006) explained the problem that faced Japanese occupational therapists in trying to use concepts developed in Western countries within the context of Japanese culture. He stated:

> By trying to fit theory and assessments based on cultural patterns so remarkably different from those of the Japanese, a professional crisis was evident. The concepts of imported occupational therapy and theories have been left largely unreconciled to indigenous experience of reality. They are written in a foreign symbolic system (language) with many concepts having no direct equivalent in the Japanese lexicon. Their definitions are reduced to straight translations that are rote memorized, having the form of occupational therapy in the West but lacking meaning and the power to inform and guide a meaningful, valued practice. (p. 117)

Although such cross-cultural dilemmas are made explicit in Iwama's work, he posited that similar cross-cultural challenges exist wherever the cultural norms that underpin the culture of Western occupational therapy, as embodied in its contemporary models, fail to resonate with the cultures of clients and with occupational therapists.

Iwama (2006) illustrated the problem of cultural translation of Western theory into Japanese culture through an anecdote about running a workshop for Japanese occupational therapists on occupational theory. He found that, at the end of the workshop, the participants did not understand the theories any better than when they had started. He gradually became aware that this workshop was probably one of many that the participants had attended in an earnest attempt to understand occupational theory. Due to the pervasive experience by Japanese members of the occupational therapy profession of difficulty in understanding the theoretical concepts underpinning occupational therapy, Iwama began to think that the problem might lie in the cultural relevance of the theory, rather than problems in the participants. As he stated:

> Having no tangible narratives or models that held meaning within their own cultural understandings, Japanese therapists were reporting a certain degree of frustration regarding the lack of philosophical and ideological guidelines that defined occupational therapy in a comprehensible way. Their identities as occupational therapists were being jeopardized as they lacked meaningful theory that would aid them in explaining the scope and boundaries of their practice. (p. 119)

This awareness provided the impetus for the development of a culturally relevant occupational therapy theory. Believing that, as occupational therapy had existed in Japan for 35 years, there must be some sort of tacit conceptual basis to the "forms of practice that were observable on the surface" (p. 120), Iwama approached a group of Japanese practitioners and made the suggestion (which he claimed "seemed audacious at the time" (p. 119)) that they develop their own model. This process resulted in the development of the Kawa model.

Iwama (2006) claimed that three concepts fundamental to Western understandings of occupational therapy were critically challenged in the development of the Kawa model. These were "the central incumbency of the individual, a tacit understanding of humans as occupational beings, [and] occupation typified as the interface between self and environment" (p. 139). Each assumption is discussed.

## CENTRALITY OF THE INDIVIDUAL

First, like many other Asian cultures, Japan is a collectivist culture in which the concept of a self separate to surrounding phenomena such as other people, plants, animals and inanimate structures like rocks is completely foreign. In explaining the difference between this assumption and the Western worldview that shapes much of occupational therapy's perspective, Iwama (2006) described a Western view as an "existential perspective" (p. 142) in which the individual self is the focal point. This existential perspective is evident in terms such as *person-centred* and *client-centred* (where client is conceptualized as an individual). These terms are commonly used in occupational therapy discourse to emphasize the value placed on people, as distinct from bodies – hence contrasting a holistic perspective with a biomedical one. However, they also attest to the focus on individuals that is paramount in Western cultures.

In contrast, collectivist cultures view each individual as just one of many different elements that combine in a mutually influencing way to constitute life. The collective is the focal point of this cultural view and harmony within the collective becomes the goal, compared to individual mastery of the environment in an individualist culture. Iwama used the term *decentralized self* to refer to this concept of the self as "embedded in groups and inseparable from nature and environment" (p. 39). Iwama (2006) explained that the decentralized concept of self derives from the "East Asian cosmological myth or worldview, which configures the universe and all of its elements (including deities, natural flora and fauna, animate and inanimate matter) in one inseparable whole" (p. 41).

## OCCUPATIONAL BEINGS

The second assumption challenged by Iwama is the concept of humans as occupational beings, which is central to much occupational therapy discourse. In relation to this premise, Iwama raises two issues for consideration. The first is whether humans are 'occupational' by nature. The second deals with the doing, being and becoming framework proposed by Wilcock (1998) that flows from the assumption that humans are occupational beings.

Regarding the assertion that humans are occupational by nature, occupational science concluded from empirical research that humans had a biological need for occupation. This assumption underpins the notion that engagement in occupation enhances health and well-being, in that people need to do things in order to maintain their health and well-being. This assumption has been a core principle in occupational therapy theory since its foundation. For example, a well-known quote is that "man [sic], through the use of his hands as they are energized by mind and will, can influence the state of his own health" (Reilly, 1962).

However, Iwama (2006) proposed that the concept of humans as occupational beings is based on an existential, rather than collectivist, understanding of humans and, therefore, might not have relevance for collectivist cultures. He explained that, from an existential perspective, humans obtain mastery over the environment by acting upon it. They exercise their personal agency. That is, through engagement in occupation, they can be agents of change in the environment. The concept of mastery of the environment has been a central concept in occupational therapy theory since the early days of the profession.

This type of association between personal agency and action and health and well-being does not have relevance from a collectivist perspective, in that personal agency does not logically lead to enhanced health and well-being through mastery over the environment. As Iwama explained, "In the Japanese collective experience, more than the self, the group in which one holds membership is agent" (p. 51). In a collectivist society, persons and the environment are not juxtaposed and understood as separate entities, but are all parts of the collective whole. Therefore, to enhance the health of the whole, individuals need to act *within* environments rather than *on* them. As the context within which one lives is part of the self, it makes little sense to attempt to maintain mastery over something that is, by definition, a part of your self. Instead, health and well-being are associated with creating and maintaining harmony between people and the contexts in which they live. As Iwama (2006) explained, "states of well-being are contingent on human and natural relations... harmony between self and others and between selves and nature, forms the cornerstones on which 'security', belonging and states of well-being among Japanese people ultimately rests. The necessity to belong and the persistent drive for harmony form the basis to Japanese 'collectivism'." (p. 116.) Thus, wellness is the result of harmony and balance between all elements in a person's life.

Emerging from the assumption that humans are occupational beings is the Doing, Being and Becoming framework. In this framework, Wilcock (1998) proposed that "*doing* well, well-*being* and *becoming* what people are best fitted to become is essential to health" (p. 255). However, Iwama (2006) demonstrated the culturally specific nature of this framework by articulating its lack of relevance to Japanese culture. He proposed that, to be more appropriate to Japanese culture, the order of the concepts should be belonging, being and doing (rather than commencing with doing then moving to being and becoming) because Japanese people are primarily accountable to their social relationships. As he stated, "matters of identity and meaning are ascribed in collective rather than in introspective processes... Roles are bestowed by the group and received by the individual, for no individual is considered greater than the collective. And once the role is made explicit, the self emerges to carry out the mandate of the collective." (p. 52.) Thus, in a collectivist society, belonging precedes and directs doing.

## RECONCEPTUALIZING OCCUPATION

The third assumption critiqued by the Kawa model is that occupation is typified as the interface between self and the environment. As the first two assumptions have demonstrated, an existential approach assumes that the person and environment are separate and that occupation is the means by which persons can act upon the environment to master it. However, when moving away from this perspective, occupation and its purpose require reconceptualizing. From a collectivist perspective, individual action flows from one's place in the group and is a consequence of belonging, rather than the means by which one interacts with the environment and through which one self-actualizes. Ones sense of self is developed by knowing and experiencing one's place within the context of the group rather than through individual action. Therefore, individual action is determined by the needs of the collective and engaged in by the individual as a consequence of his or her place within the group. Thus, occupation is not the means by which one masters the environment but a consequence of one's place in the group.

This difference has important implications for a conceptualization of occupation. In current occupational therapy discourse, occupation is defined as action that is meaningful to the person. In an existential culture, human action becomes meaningful to the individual when it relates to individual goals, interests and values. In a collectivist culture, human action becomes meaningful to the individual when it serves the function of fulfilling the requirements of the collective and sustains the individual's position within the group. As Iwama (2006) stated, "In Japanese society, *doing* is important but may not mean much when separated from the social context in which it occurs and from which meaning is derived" (p. 116). Therefore, the contextualized meanings of occupations have to be understood.

The difference in these perspectives is highlighted when considering the assessment and goal setting tools that are used in occupational therapy practice. Because of the association made between (meaningful) occupation and individual goal setting, eliciting and establishing client-centred goals is the primary way that priorities are set within client-centred occupational therapy practice. However, to determine meaningful occupation within a collectivist culture, assessments probably need to commence with an understanding of belonging rather than goals. Such an understanding would then allow the occupational therapist to work with the client to determine what kind of occupation could be used to support the client's sense of belonging.

Another aspect of Japanese society that differs from Western cultures is a different orientation to time. In general, Western cultures are future oriented. This is evident in occupational therapy practice through the emphasis on goal setting when aiming to be client-centred. The assumption is that mastery of the environment is achieved by achieving goals. However, Japanese society is characterized by a temporal orientation that is located in the present. The implication for occupational therapy practice is that, rather than using therapeutic activity or occupations to meet goals (for the future), the process of therapy itself becomes most important.

## DEVELOPMENT OF THE MODEL

The Kawa model was developed by occupational therapists, educators and students in Western Japan using a naturalistic research methodology that combined heuristic research and (modified) Grounded Theory. They used these qualitative research methods to "mine original concepts germane to their experience and interpretation of Japanese occupational therapy" (Iwama,

2006, p. 120). They aimed to develop a conceptual model that was "derived from Japanese subjects, in Japanese language, using Japanese concepts and metaphors having high contextual meaning" (p. 120). Iwama claimed that the Kawa model was one of the first of its kind in Asia where the tendency has been to import their theory from the Western world.

A group of 20 participants, representing a diversity of clinical practice backgrounds, met monthly in focus groups for approximately 6 hours per session over a 2½-year period. In total, the group met over 50 times. The only inclusion criteria for these groups were that participants "had an interest in occupational therapy theory and desired to participate in making their clinical practice theoretically clearer" (p. 121). While grounded theory, which is widely used in Japan, provided the overall structure for the research, culturally relevant modifications were made to the process of collecting data. For example, as the social behaviour of people in Japanese society is influenced by their place within the social hierarchy, they are likely to defer to the opinions of senior members of the group. In order to minimize such hierarchical influences on the data that were collected, three modifications were made. These were: making expectations clear that senior members of the group would both allow and encourage junior members to express their opinions, using smaller sub groups to enhance the expression of a range of group members, and using a range of data collection methods such as writing responses on cards and collectively developing drawn diagrams that did not rely on verbal expression in the context of the larger group.

A number of questions were used to generate data. Initially, two open-ended questions were used to focus the discussion. These were: "How do you as Japanese occupational therapists conceive of the concepts of health and disability and illness?" and "What, if there is any, role or relation does occupational therapy have with these concepts?" These questions were used to explore the participants' perspectives of the meaning of occupational therapy in Japan. These questions were deemed important, as the identity crisis that occupational therapists appeared to feel was observed to be widespread. Subsequently, the general line of enquiry explored the question, "What is the meaning of Japanese occupational therapy?" Other questions were used to guide the enquiry more specifically and provide more structure for those who required it to complete the task. These included: "What is your role in Japanese society?"; "What do you do (in regard to intervention) and why?"; "Who are your clients?"; "What are you concerned with in your work?"; "How do you (Japanese OTs) define and regard 'health', 'disability'?" (pp. 126–127). Data were recorded in the form of photographs of the sorted and assembled data, notes taken by participants were logged as data, and some sessions were videotaped.

Iwama (2006) described in detail the standard Grounded Theory process of analyzing the data inductively by coding the data using the early steps of open coding and axial coding whereby data are "fractured" (p. 127) into minute sections and then combined into groupings of connected categories, respectively. Iwama remarked that, when explaining the codes produced in the axial coding stage, the participants explained each code in terms of its situational context. He suggested that "situational relativism was apparent throughout the procedure and highlighted the importance that context or 'ba' plays as an important factor in the interpretation and judgment of realities for these Japanese therapists" (p. 127). Iwama (2006) also commented on participants' preference, when asked about the meaning of occupational therapy, to emphasize 'life' and 'life force'.

Through the processes of grouping the data, five tentative thematic categories were developed. These were (Iwama, 2006, p. 128):

- Life flow and health
- Environmental factors (social, 'ba', physical barriers)
- Life circumstances and problems
- Personal assets and liabilities
- Occupational therapy intervention

The final phase of data analysis in Grounded Theory is selective coding. In undertaking this process, in which a 'central concept' is selected and related to the other categories, it became clear that no concept could be identified as more central than the others. Instead, all the concepts were linked and considered to be mutually influencing. As Iwama (2006) explained, "This configuration and structure could be described as a dynamic rubric in which a disruption or change in magnitude and quality of any one concept would affect the magnitude and quality of all of the other concepts." (p. 129.) He also described how, prior to the selective coding phase of data analysis, one participant's proposal that these five concepts and their inter relatedness could be explained better through the use of a river metaphor had been met with resounding acceptance by the whole group. This unanimous consent led to the use of the river metaphor, which appeared to be more consistent with a society "whose cosmologies are based on a naturalistic paradigm and whose ideations of humans are constructively inseparable from nature, society and deities" (p. 129) than a diagram consisting of boxes with arrows to show their relationships.

The river metaphor clearly resonated with the Japanese participants during the development of the conceptual model because it had specific cultural meanings. Iwama provided a quote from one of the Japanese research leaders in which she explained the central and symbolic place the river has in Japanese society and culture. After saying that, given the rich meaning of rivers in Japanese culture, it would seem superfluous to state that rivers are metaphors for life, she wrote:

> The river evokes in itself a very rich picture of mental imagery for a Japanese.
> A projection method developed in Japan called 'fukei kousei hou' also uses the river
> as 'a metaphor of unconscious flow'. By looking at this holistic picture of our clients
> and by using such images that flow right deep inside our hearts, we may sympathize
> with their komari (problems) as people who live just like ourselves, otherwise we may
> understand their komari as something that happens to someone else somewhere in life.
> The clients that we treat and support are living persons. An approach without such
> sympathy carries the risk of being superficial and an affront to our clients. (p. 141)

In this quote, she emphasized not only the rich cultural meaning of rivers in Japan but also that this kind of metaphor would help occupational therapists to understand problems as human problems that touch us all.

Iwama (2006) emphasized that using the image of water flowing in a river to represent life flow also refocuses occupational therapy on facilitating life flow rather than increasing an individual's self-efficacy. In explaining the relationship between life flow and the important concept of occupation, Iwama stated:

> *Occupation is reconceptualised to be the flow of water in this river. Without water flowing, there can be no river. Without occupation, in the context of this cosmological view of all elements in a frame or context inextricably connected, there can be no life. In this way, one's own or one's group's occupations are interwoven and connected to the occupation of others. Well-being is a collective phenomenon. Occupational therapy's purpose in this metaphorical representation of human being, then, is to enable and enhance life flow – a flow that encompasses self and context. (p. 144)*

## USE OF THE MODEL IN PRACTICE

One of the ways that the Kawa model appears to differ from many other occupational therapy models is its use in practice. The majority of occupational therapy models have been developed as theoretical perspectives that are used to guide occupational therapists in their conceptualization of humans and human occupation and performance and their consequent collection, organization and integration of information. As such, the primary role of conceptual models is to guide and shape the perspectives of occupational therapists. This is an important function as it assists the profession to define its scope and focus and to articulate the uniqueness of its perspective on phenomena such as health and well-being. As a consequence, these conceptual models assist individual occupational therapists to define confidently the scope and focus of their practice in their local practice context and articulate their particular perspective. However, it is conceivable that the conceptual models that were developed were never intended to be shared with clients or other professionals. Instead, their value lies in providing an organizing structure to guide the practice of occupational therapists and a foundation from which they can use their interpersonal and professional skills to work with clients and professionals.

In contrast, the Kawa model was designed to be used as a basis for discussion with clients. In explaining this approach and with reference to a more traditional approach to theory, Iwama stated, "We may claim to be enacting client-centred practice, yet the clients' narratives are ultimately reduced, organized and made sense of through the structure, language and explanatory principles of our professional models and theories" (p. 159). In using the Kawa model, the client narrative is preserved as a whole and used as a basis for discussion.

In discussing using the Kawa model in practice, Iwama (2006) stated:

> *There is not one 'right' way to use and apply the Kawa model. The Kawa is a metaphor for life. The right way is realized when the model is adapted and used as a vehicle to illuminate the client's narrative for his or her life at a certain place and point in time. The Kawa model's ultimate form will be determined by the unique qualities of the client and the occupational therapy frame. (pp. 162–163)*

In emphasizing that there is no right way to use the model, Iwama also stressed that the metaphor of a river might not be the most appropriate metaphor to use for a particular client and an alternative metaphor can be used.

The two principles that guide its use are that it honour the client (and their cultural context) and that the occupational therapist trust "that the client's narrative will emerge through a process of enabling him or her to do so" (p. 160).

While originally designed in the context of Japanese society, the Kawa model has been presented as a model that should be used and changed as appropriate to other cultural and situational contexts. As the only current occupational therapy model to address collectivist cultures, it represents a departure from traditional ways of thinking about human occupation and is likely to provide the catalyst for further development of other models appropriate to collectivist cultures. Recent reports (Iwama, 2009) on the applicability of the Kawa model suggest that the model carries promise for use in individualist cultures as well.

The process of using the Kawa model in practice revolves around the drawing of a river (or other) diagram (or another form of creation of an appropriate metaphor). In doing this, the first decision should be about who will draw the diagram. At times, this might be the client and at other times it might be the occupational therapist in discussion with the client. In many cases, the client is not limited to the individual but may consist of family members, and/or others who represent the client's best interests. This is particularly seen in contexts of occupational therapy with children, people with dementia, persons with intellectual challenges, various mental health conditions, etc.

In summary, the Kawa model was developed by a group of Japanese occupational therapists in order to develop an occupational therapy model that was culturally appropriate for them. Therefore, the model does not purport to be relevant in its original form to all cultures. Instead, occupational therapists are encouraged to use metaphors (either of the river or something else if that works better) that have cultural significance to the people with whom they are working. In presenting the Kawa model, Iwama (2006) explained the cultural context that it aimed to address. It is important that, in developing an understanding of the model, people understand the many cultural concepts that underpin it, such as the decentralized self within a collectivist culture. Unlike many other occupational therapy models, practitioners are encouraged to adapt the model for use in their local context.

See Box 7.1.

---

**BOX 7.1  Kawa model memory aid**

**Creation of the client's river**
Who (a person or collective) or what (organization, community, professional teams, etc.) is the client?

How will the client's narrative be created? e.g. Will it be a river diagram? Who will draw it?

In what context will it be discussed? How will I elicit the client's own words and perspectives and their descriptions of their circumstances?

**Elements of the river**
How are the elements of the client's river depicted at the moment?

■ River walls and floor

■ Rocks

■ Driftwood

■ Water flow (where is this flowing at the moment?)

What is the river's history? How has the river been organized at different times?

**Significance of the elements**
What is the importance (relative size and shape) and meaning of each of the elements of the river to the client?

How do they affect the flow of the water? (in the present and past)

**Change in the river**
What could be changed (if anything could or needs to be) to increase the flow in the river?

If something changed in the river, how would this affect other elements?

What aspects of the river need to stay the same?

What would the occupational therapy contribution be to this change?

How would we know if the changes in the river were useful ones for the client?

---

# CONCLUSION

The Kawa model was developed by a group of Japanese occupational therapists because of the difficulty they were having understanding many of the occupational therapy concepts that they were 'importing' from Western countries. Therefore, the focus of this model of practice is culturally relevant occupational therapy.

The model uses the metaphor of a river to represent life flow. The various elements of the river are used to represent different aspects of life in the context of a particular society. The river metaphor was chosen as it had particular meaning to Japanese people. Throughout the major text, Iwama emphasized the need to use the model in a way that is relevant culturally for both occupational therapists and their clients. Therefore, the metaphor of a river should only be used if it has cultural relevance, otherwise different metaphors should be selected.

In discussing the model, Iwama explained the nature of Japanese society, with its hierarchical structure and collective nature. Iwama also critiqued many accepted occupational therapy concepts relating to the nature of humans and occupation and explained how embedded in Western views of the world they were. For example, the primacy of belonging over doing in Japanese culture was explained. In these discussions, important cultural concepts were presented such as the decentralized self, the East Asian cosmological myth, and a Japanese cultural understanding of the world. Despite its purported benefits to practical application, the Kawa model's most important contribution to the discourse on theory in occupational therapy may be in its subtle influence on how power is structured and enacted in occupational therapeutic relationships. The Kawa model aims to privilege the unique narratives of each client, allowing the client to ultimately name the concepts and explain the principles that connect them. Whereas the conventional pattern of model use is for the theorist or therapist to create the concepts and principles of a model and apply them universally to all clients, the Kawa model aims to reverse this familiar power dynamic, and make the client's unique story of their day-to-day realities the centre of occupational therapy's concern.

The Kawa model is the most recently developed of the models of practice presented in this book. The purpose of the river metaphor is to facilitate discussion that leads to an understanding of the client's unique circumstances and needs. Unlike many other models, the Kawa model was devised to be used with clients. Despite being a relatively new model, its development and application to a variety of cultures appears to be rapid and broad.

## MAJOR WORKS

Iwama, M., 2006. The Kawa model: Culturally relevant occupational therapy. Churchill Livingstone, Edinburgh.

Iwama, M., 2006. The Kawa model: Culturally relevant occupational therapy. Churchill Livingstone, Edinburgh.

Iwama, M., 2009. The Kawa Model; the power of culturally responsive occupational therapy. Disabil. Rehabil. 31 (14), 1125–1135.

Reilly, M., 1962. Occupational therapy can be one of the great ideas of 20th century medicine. Am. J. Occup. Ther. 16 (1), 1–9.

Wilcock, A., 1998. Reflections on doing, being and becoming. Can. J. Occup. Ther. 65 (5), 248–257.

Kawa model

# Occupational therapy concepts

**8**

## CHAPTER CONTENTS

This chapter discusses how models of practice illustrate the trends in concepts and priorities in occupational therapy over time. Occupational therapy is a profession that exists within the broader context of societies. Consequently, the roles and perspectives of occupational therapy will differ from country to country, place to place, and at different historical times. The models of practice presented in this book largely reflect the perspectives of occupational therapy in Western countries. Other excellent texts such as *Occupational Therapy without Borders* (Kronenberg et al., 2005) explore the perspectives of occupational therapy from non-Western countries. However, these perspectives have not been specifically included in this book because there have not been many models of practice emanating from non-Western countries.

The only model included here that originated from work done in a non-Western country is the Kawa model (Iwama, 2006). Such models are important as they not only bring a novel and different perspective on occupational therapy, but their emergence from a different worldview also illuminates the cultural features of contemporary occupational therapy thought, theory and practices. Such alternative models reveal the cultural nature of the profession's core concepts as well as the context of experience through which its ideas of occupation are interpreted. They can highlight how occupational therapy makes sense of and privileges the individual as the central concern through which occupations are interpreted, understands the relationship between individuals and environments, and conceptualizes occupation. Awareness of and reflection upon these revelations can bring to debate how power is constructed and exercised in occupational therapy and is inherent in values and procedures such as client centredness as well as in important processes such as engagement and enablement. It will be interesting to see how this relatively recent

**179**

acknowledgement of the Western-centric nature of occupational therapy theory plays out in the future. For example, it is already the case that many of the more recent versions of models of practice from Western countries are incorporating into their models consideration of the collective nature of some cultural perspectives and including concepts of cultural safety. We might also see more models of practice originating in non-Western countries in the future.

This book presented a historical approach to models of practice. When understanding and using models in practice, it is important to have a sense of the purpose for which they were developed. Typically, models are developed to fulfil a perceived need. Often this relates to the surrounding context, whereby the model identifies the limitations of the current views and proposes alternative or extended views. Three examples are provided.

The first example is the Model of Human Occupation (MOHO) (Kielhofner, 1985, 1995, 2002, 2008). The first edition of MOHO was produced because of the perceived need to provide a structure that made explicit the relationships between the multitude of concepts generated within the occupational behaviour tradition. Occupational behaviour was developed by Mary Reilly because of her perception of the limitations of a biomedical model of health (mechanistic and reductionist in approach, characteristic of medicine and dominating health in the 1960s and 70s) and of occupational therapy's alignment with this. As this critique of a mechanical view of persons was central to both occupational behaviour and MOHO, it is not surprising that the limitations of a mechanistic view of humans (upon which biomedicine is based) remained a theme throughout all four editions of MOHO.

Another example is the Kawa model (Iwama, 2006). This was developed because of the perception that a Western-centric understanding pervaded occupational therapy theory and the difficulty occupational therapists in Japan had in understanding many occupational therapy concepts (because of their poor cultural relevance). It also aimed to fill a gap in understanding diversity of cultural perspectives such as collective cultures. Because of its cultural emphasis and critique of Western-centric occupational therapy concepts, it appears that the Kawa model has a broader appeal than just in Japan. Because of this emphasis on culture, it is presented as a model that needs to be changed and adapted as appropriate to the cultural context in which it is being used. This is quite different from many of the other models of practice, which encourage faithfulness to the model as it has been published. The same level of consistency is also important when using assessments requiring validation that were developed from a particular model. Thus, many other models rely on their concepts being used consistently, rather than being changed and adapted for the particular setting in which they are being used. As the issue of cultural specificity of theoretical material (and the assessments that derive from them) becomes more apparent, we may see a fundamental shift in how models are critiqued, constructed and adapted for use across diverse practice contexts.

A third example is the Canadian Model of Occupational Performance and Engagement (CMOP-E) (Townsend & Polatajko, 2007). This model was presented within a text that claimed in its title to be *Advancing an occupational therapy vision for health, well-being and justice through occupation*. In that text, the model was changed from the original Canadian Model of Occupational

Performance (CMOP) model to include engagement because of the claim that the concept of engagement in occupation does not necessarily require performance. In this way, one perceived gap that this model aimed to address was the limitations that the concept of occupational performance placed on an occupational therapy perspective. The model also addresses the concern that some individuals, groups and populations (or subpopulations) do not have equal opportunities for occupational engagement. Consequently, it includes aims and processes that target the enhancement of equity of engagement that promote justice. Certainly, the concept of occupational justice is not explicitly addressed in any of the other models to date.

Local needs were also the impetus for the development of some of the other models covered in this book. In many cases, specific models were created to guide the development and implementation of a specific occupational therapy curriculum. In these cases, particular staff undertook the role of developing the model and they often then remained responsible for its further development. Other models were developed on behalf of national occupational therapy bodies.

## USING MODELS IN PRACTICE

In this book, we presented models of practice as resources that can be used in and should *serve* practice. We aimed to present each model in an objective way, describing both the current version and placing it (and any previous versions) within a historical context. The purpose of doing this is to provide practitioners with a resource to use to support and enhance their practice. The specific situation in which the occupational therapist is located will shape his or her need for and use of models of practice. By presenting a brief overview of each model, we anticipate that practitioners will be in a strong position to evaluate the potential utility of each model in their specific practice context. By understanding the main features of the model as well as the context within which it was developed and the gap or purpose it aimed to fill, practitioners can make comparisons with the demands of their own roles, the needs of their own clients, and the nature of their organizational and social context. These comparisons can then inform their choices about which model/s to use and how. We aimed to make the process of comparison easier by approaching each model in a similar way (main concepts and definitions of terms and a historical description of the model's development) and providing a single-page memory aid.

In addition to providing an overview of a range of different occupational therapy models, we also provided a model for understanding how occupational therapists reason within specific contexts and how they turn their thinking into action. The various different models can help to shape this thinking, perceiving and acting, depending on the demands of the role that practitioners are fulfilling. For example, if they are working directly with individual clients with a particular type of need, they might choose a model that helps them to understand that need (possibly by providing the right amount of detail). Their role might involve designing programmes for groups of people or they might be providing training to direct service providers. In such cases, other models might provide more support for them in that role.

As well as evaluating the potential utility of each model of practice to a particular practice setting, occupational therapists also need to consider how well each model resonates with their own particular professional reasoning styles. By that we mean that some models will align better than others with the ways a particular occupational therapist understands occupational therapy and the aspects of occupational therapy that he or she might particularly emphasize. For example, someone who emphasizes the role of the environment in their understanding of occupation is likely to find one of the ecological models most useful, someone who is more interested in understanding how the body works is likely to find one of the occupational performance models of greatest use, and someone who is especially concerned with social equity might find the CMOP-E of particular use.

Professionals can use models of practice like a lens through which to create meaning in practice. Practice is complex and rarely presents to the practitioner in an organized or patterned way. Instead, it is the professional's job to make meaning and order from what can appear to be a chaotic mess. It is their job to organize information into meaningful patterns and clusters. Each model provides a lens (or window, to use our original metaphor) through which to see practice. As with all lenses (or windows), they frame what people see (and don't see), they guide them in their interpretation of what they see, and they magnify some aspects of the situation more than others. This vision that they develop with the assistance of models can inform what action they will consider taking.

## TRENDS IN OCCUPATIONAL THERAPY THEORY

### A RENAISSANCE OF OCCUPATION

A major trend that has occurred in occupational therapy theory is the acceptance of the centrality of occupation. Kielhofner (2009) stated that occupation had been a unifying concept in occupational therapy following the mechanistic period in which the profession lost its identity as a unified whole. Whiteford et al. (2000) noted that occupational therapy had undergone a renaissance of occupation, in that it was returning to its founding roots.

However, the concept of occupation in occupational therapy has changed over time. The term was used during the founding period of the profession to refer to occupying time and having meaningful things to do. During the mechanistic period, occupation was approached in a very technical way in that it was primarily used as a tool to achieve specific goals. During that time, it was generally understood as a means to an (therapeutic) end. The models (or versions) in the 1990s primarily emphasized occupational performance, in which the *performance* of occupation was the primary consideration.

More recently, the concept of performance is being explored and critiqued as the major focus of occupational therapy and broader understandings (than performance) are being accepted. For example, Baum and Christiansen (2005) placed occupational performance and participation (rather than just occupational performance) at the centre of the

Person-Environment-Occupation-Performance (PEOP) model, and CMOP-E included the concept of engagement rather than just occupational performance. In explaining this change (from the CMOP), Townsend and Polatajko (2007) provided a narrative about a severely disabled young man participating in marathons and triathlons with his father without 'performing' these occupations. This trend away from occupational performance as an end in itself (i.e. it can be a means to participation) might also align with the increasing influence of the International Classification of Functioning, Disability and Health (ICF), published by the World Health Organization (2001), in the broader health field. In the ICF, activities and participation are major categories. It might also relate to increased awareness that the notions of independence and the importance of individual action are Western assumptions and are not necessarily relevant or valued in other cultures.

At the time of publication of this book, the return to or renaissance of occupation was well embedded in current occupational therapy thinking. The link between occupation and social roles (or occupational roles) was also very much emphasized. That is, the meaning and purpose of occupation was acknowledged as integral to people's participation in the society in which they live. There was also increasing acknowledgement that the structure of the society in which a person lives may advantage or disadvantage that person and that many people in their societies have unequal access to health services and resources. Consequently, occupational therapists' roles were increasingly seen as working with groups and populations, rather than just individuals, and might include activities other than direct service, such as policy development and advocacy.

## IMPORTANCE OF CONTEXT

A second pervasive trend in occupational therapy in recent times has been a greater acknowledgement of and focus on the context-specific nature of engagement in occupation. While the concept of the environment has always been an important aspect of occupational therapy thinking, the trend in earlier models was to focus on the person. This was evident in the concept of performance components, which were a major feature of the occupational performance models. In these various occupational performance models, the performance components were divided into different constellations of motor, sensory, cognitive, perceptual, social and psychological components. It is likely that this trend aligned with the primary biomedical approach that dominated health until quite late in the twentieth century. In a biomedical approach, the causes of problems and ill-health are understood to be located within the body. The assumption is that, by locating the cause, an intervention could be used to target or 'cure' the problem. In occupational therapy, this approach generally translated into analyzing functional problems in order to devise appropriate interventions. Because occupational therapy has always been more of a biopsychosocial practice, this analysis included an understanding of the person's subjective experience as well as the analysis of their body's capacities. Some of the models of practice and editions published in the 1990s emphasized this biopsychosocial approach in particular.

However, the occupational therapy models of practice also show a trend away from a primarily intrapersonal perspective to a focus on the person in context. Towards the end of the twentieth century, a range of models of practice presented an ecological approach, in which context was a primary focus. The two models at the time that particularly took such an approach were Person-Environment-Occupation (PEO) (Law et al., 1996) and Ecology of Human Performance (EHP) (Dunn et al., 1994). In addition, the interconnectedness of person and environment is evident in the Occupational Performance Model (Australia) (OPMA) (Chapparo & Ranka, 1997) through its concepts of internal and external environments. Since these major publications in the mid 1990s, the concepts of person, environment and occupation have become incorporated into much of mainstream occupational therapy thinking. It appears that this ecological understanding of occupation has manifest in current occupational therapy models and versions of models through the increased focus on occupation in context.

This contextualized understanding is often presented through the concepts of person and environment, which are understood to be mutually influencing. In contrast to the ecological models of the 1990s, current models tend to separate person and environment into two interactive components rather than seeing them as inseparable. The fact that many current versions of occupational therapy models of practice present occupation as the bridge or vehicle by which person and environment are connected, attests to the separation of these concepts. In some models of practice, occupation is conceptualized as the means by which people obtain mastery over the environment (e.g. Occupational Adaptation). Other models conceptualize a more reciprocal contribution of person and environment (i.e. one is not necessarily considered to be mastering the other). The PEOP model (Baum & Christiansen, 2005) provides an example of the mutually influencing relationship between the person and environment. In the diagrammatic representation of that model, the person and environment are presented as two even circles that touch and are overlapped evenly by occupation, performance, occupational performance and participation. The more recent versions of MOHO also present the person and environment as mutually influencing and linked by occupation.

In contrast, ecological models assumed a transactive or inseparable relationship between person and environment. In such an approach, occupation might be conceptualized quite differently from those that separate person and environment. As there is no gap to bridge between occupation and person, there is no need to conceptualize occupation as a bridge that spans this gap. While the two ecological models presented in this book both originated from North America, the only current occupational therapy model of practice that takes this kind of ecological model is the Kawa model.

Iwama (2003) questioned the conception of the role of occupation in providing the vehicle through which people and environments interact. He expressed the view that in collectivist societies, people first belong and then act (i.e. their doing flows from their belonging). They are a part of the environment and their place within that environment shapes and provides the impetus for action. In the image of the river, the life flow that could be understood to represent the person is shaped and shapes the river sides and bottom and the various rocks and driftwood that lie in the river. People act (occupation) according to the constellation of factors that make up the river at the time. Their action is shaped by and cannot be separated from the social and physical context in which they live.

A review of the models of practice in this book shows that occupational therapy's current understanding of the relationships among person, environment and occupation appear generally to be interactive rather than transactive or ecological (with the exception of the Kawa model). This is in contrast to the trend in the 1990s. It may be that the renaissance of occupation has contributed to this trend, in that occupational therapy has been concerned primarily with conceptualizing and articulating the nature of occupation rather than with the interconnectedness of all three concepts. As occupation is less likely to occupy the central place in an ecological understanding of person, environment and occupation (where the three are not separate entities), it may be that an ecological understanding of their relationship is less consistent with the idea that occupation is the core of occupational therapy. The issue of the relationships among person, environment and occupation and occupation as the core of the profession provides a tension for the profession. It will be interesting to see how the profession addresses this tension in the future.

## CONCLUSION

Nine occupational therapy models of practice were reviewed in this book. Taking a historical approach to these models highlights some of the trends and changes in occupational therapy theory and practice since the early 1980s. Readers are encouraged to refer to other texts for a more complete history of the profession and its ideas and for detailed descriptions of each model of practice. To this end, a list of the major publications has been included for each model of practice.

This review of the major models of occupational therapy practice since that time shows a trend away from the biomedical perspective that influenced health substantially from the 1960s, through an emphasis on a more biopsychosocial approach in the 1990s, towards a renewed focus on occupation from the end of the twentieth century. Within this period of centring on occupation, there has also been a move from a focus on occupational performance to broader concepts of occupation that include participation, engagement and justice. As models of practice embed the important theoretical concepts of occupational therapy, they are a good way of understanding the primary focus of occupational therapy at different times.

Models of practice are also developed to assist occupational therapists in putting theory into practice. In this book we have presented the models as tools that should serve practice. As professional practice requires decision-making and action under conditions of uncertainty, readers are encouraged to consider both their own ways of reasoning and the practice context within which they are reasoning and acting when making decisions about the potential use of models in their practice.

Baum, C., Christiansen, C., 2005. Person-Environment-Occupation-Performance: An occupation-based framework for practice. In: Christiansen, C.H., Baum, C.M., Bass-Haugen, J. (Eds.), Occupational therapy: Performance, participation, and well-being, third ed. Slack, Thorofare, NJ, pp. 243–259.

Chapparo, C., Ranka, J., 1997. OPM: Occupational Performance Model (Australia), Monograph 1. Occupational Performance Network, Lidcombe, NSW.

Dunn, W., Brown, C., McGuigan, A., 1994. The ecology of human performance: A framework for considering the effect of context. Am. J. Occup. Ther. 48 (7), 595–607.

Iwama, M., 2003. The issue is…toward culturally relevant epistemologies in occupational therapy. Am. J. Occup. Ther. 57 (5), 217–223.

Iwama, M., 2006. The Kawa model: Culturally relevant occupational therapy. Churchill Livingstone, Edinburgh.

Kielhofner, G. (Ed.), 1985. A model of human occupation: Theory and application. Williams & Wilkins, Baltimore, MD.

Kielhofner, G., 1995. A model of human occupation: Theory and application, second ed. Williams & Wilkins, Baltimore, MD.

Kielhofner, G., 2002. A model of human occupation: Theory and application, third ed. Lippincott Williams & Wilkins, Baltimore, MD.

Kielhofner, G., 2008. A model of human occupation: Theory and application, fourth ed. Lippincott Williams & Wilkins, Baltimore, MD.

Kielhofner, G., 2009. Conceptual foundations of occupational therapy practice, fourth ed. F.A. Davis, Philadelphia, PA.

Kronenberg, F., Simo Algado, S., Pollard, N., 2005. Occupational therapy without borders: Learning from the spirit of survivors. Churchill Livingstone, Edinburgh.

Law, M., Cooper, B., Strong, S., Stewart, D., Rigby, P., Letts, L. 1996. The Person-Environment-Occupation Model: A transactive approach to occupational performance. Can. J. Occup. Ther. 63 (1), 9–23.

Townsend, E.A., Polatajko, H.J. (Eds.), 2007. Enabling occupation II: Advancing an occupational therapy vision for health, well-being, and justice through occupation. CAOT Publications ACE, Ottawa, ON.

Whiteford, G., Townsend, E., Hocking, C., 2000. Reflections on a renaissance of occupation. Can. J. Occup. Ther. 67 (1), 324–336.

World Health Organization, 2001. ICF: International classification of functioning, disability and health (short version). World Health Organization, Geneva.

# INDEX

Note: Page numbers followed by *b* indicate boxes; *f* figures; *t* tables.

INDEX

Printed in the United States
By Bookmasters